The Best 300 Calorie Cookbook

Watching Your Weight? Discover 40 Recipes to Help You Lose Weight Fast

BY

Daniel Humphreys

Copyright 2019 Daniel Humphreys

License Notes

No part of this Book can be reproduced in any form or by any means including print, electronic, scanning or photocopying unless prior permission is granted by the author.

All ideas, suggestions and guidelines mentioned here are written for informative purposes. While the author has taken every possible step to ensure accuracy, all readers are advised to follow information at their own risk. The author cannot be held responsible for personal and/or commercial damages in case of misinterpreting and misunderstanding any part of this Book

Table of Contents

Introduction 7

Lite Bites 9

    Barbecue Chicken Wing Pizza... 10

    Cauliflower Cheese Soup with Bacon and Beer 13

    Cheese and Broccoli Egg Muffins 17

    Country Cajun Soup 20

    Crab Salad 23

    Garlic Pizza Bread 25

    Hawaiian Grilled Cheese and Bacon Sandwich............ 28

    Mediterranean Salad with Pulled Pork 31

    Minestrone Soup 34

    Mushroom, Spinach, and Cheese Quiche 38

Mains 42

    Chinese Chicken and Broccoli Stir Fry 43

    Curried Cod with Pea Slaw 46

    Green Pesto Penne with Flaked Almonds 49

    Moroccan Chicken 52

    Pan Seared Tuna with Ginger 55

    Pork Chops Italian Style 58

    Rib-Eye Steak Caprese 62

    Rosemary Chicken with Oven-Roasted Veggie 65

    Salmon Tacos with Lime Yogurt 68

    Swordfish Burgers 72

Sweet Treats 76

    Banana and Peanut Butter Cups 77

    Cheesecake Stuffed Strawberries 79

Chocolate Oatmeal Cookies 82

Cinnamon Spiced Apple Flautas 85

Coconut Macaroons 88

Cookie Dough Balls 91

Gooey Peanut Butter Bars 94

Lemon Berry Parfait 97

Peachberry Sorbet 99

Ultimate Moist Brownies 101

Smoothies 104

   Bloat Buster 105

   Cocoberry Smoothie 107

   Fruity Green Tea Smoothie 109

   Key Lime Pie Smoothie 111

   Mango Lassi 113

Mint Choc Chip Smoothie 115

Mocha Frappuccino Smoothie 117

Pumpkin Pie Smoothie 119

Tropical Breeze Smoothie 121

Vanilla Cherry Smoothie 123

Author's Afterthoughts 125

About the Author 126

Introduction

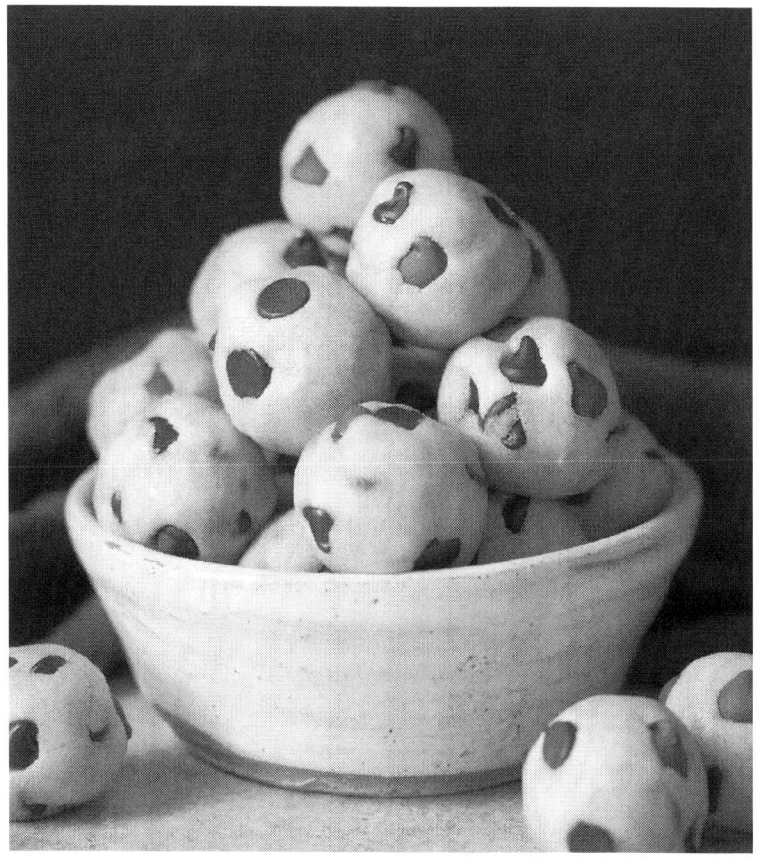

Most ready-made meals, snacks, and beverages are far more calorific than you may think and far less healthy than a homemade recipe.

A hot and creamy drink from any city coffee shop is around 400 calories, add to that a snack, and you are well on the way to consuming a whole day's calorie allowance!

A daily or even weekly menu plan is a great way to make sure that you not only stay in control of your calorie count but also eat healthy and satisfying foods.

Skipping breakfast, for instance, is the best way to get off to a bad start and can often lead to snacking on foods high in salt or sugar.

Instead, opt for an under 300 calorie, protein-packed smoothie made using fresh fruits and natural sweeteners such as honey or maple syrup.

Rather than buying pre-packed sandwiches why not pop a slice of mushroom, spinach, and cheese quiche in your lunchbox instead?

And rather than choosing a calorific bar of candy, whip up a batch of moist brownies.

The Best Under 300 Calorie Cookbook is a collection of invaluable food and drink recipes to help you count the calories, watch your weight and stay healthy.

Lite Bites

Barbecue Chicken Wing Pizza

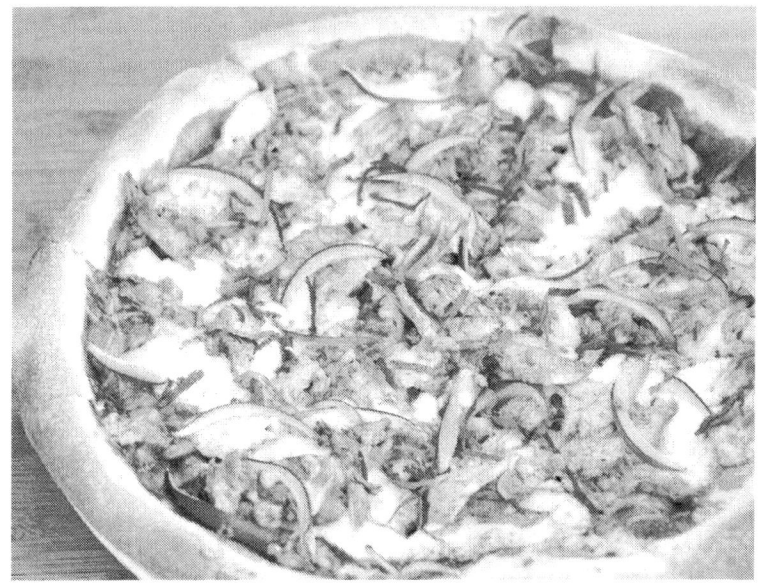

Just because you are watching your weight doesn't mean that you can't enjoy pizza. This recipe is as tasty and satisfying as any take-out version and a lot fewer calories.

Servings: 4

Total Time: 15mins

Ingredients:

- ½ cup celery (trimmed, sliced)
- 1 tbsp freshly squeezed lemon juice
- Nonstick olive oil spray
- 2 (10") ready-made whole wheat pizza crust
- ⅔ cup BBQ sauce (any brand)
- 1 cup cooked chicken (shredded)
- 2 ounces blue cheese (crumbled)

Directions:

1. Preheat the grill to moderately high heat.

2. In a bowl, combine the celery with the lemon juice and allow to marinate for 10 minutes.

3. Lightly coat each of the pizza crusts on one side only with nonstick oil.

4. Position the pizza crust, oil side facing down on the grill and heat for 2-3 minutes, until the base of the pizzas is golden.

5. Flip over and evenly spread with BBQ sauce, shredded chicken, and blue cheese.

6. Grill for 2 minutes, until the bottom of each pizza, is golden. Remove from the grill.

7. Scatter with the celery-lemon juice mixture and slice each of the pizzas into 4 and serve.

Nutrition per Serving

Cals 293 | Carbs 36g | Fat 8.5g | Fiber 8.5g | Protein 18g

Cauliflower Cheese Soup with Bacon and Beer

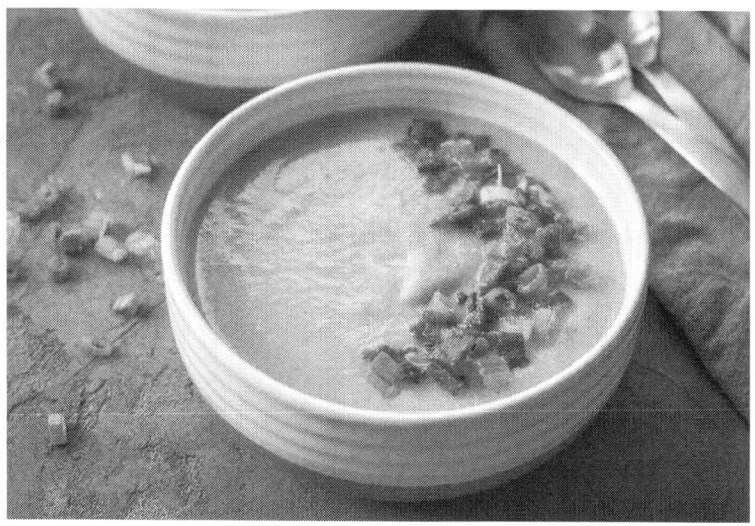

A satisfying soup for those times when you need a comforting meal and what's more your friends will beg you for this lager-infused recipe.

Servings: 6

Total Time: 40mins

Ingredients:

- Nonstick cooking spray
- 8 slices turkey bacon (chopped)
- 1 tbsp unsalted butter
- 2 cups onions (peeled, sliced)
- 3 garlic cloves (peeled, minced)
- 1 cup lager or beer (of choice)
- 3 cups chicken broth
- ½ tsp salt
- 1 cup carrots (chopped)
- 9 cups cauliflower (trimmed, chopped)
- 1 tsp mustard
- 1 tsp Worcestershire sauce
- 1 cup mature Cheddar cheese (shredded)
- Hot sauce (optional)
- Green onions (to garnish)

Directions:

1. Spritz a large pot with nonstick spray and cook the slices of turkey bacon until gently browned on both sides. Remove from the pot using a slotted spoon.

2. Add the butter along with the onions to the pot and cooked until translucent, 5-7 minutes.

3. Add the garlic and cook for an additional 60 seconds.

4. Deglaze with the lager and scrape up any bits from the bottom and sides of the pot.

5. Pour in the broth, and add the salt followed by the carrots, and cauliflower.

6. Cover the pot with a tight-fitting lid and bring to boil.

7. Continue cooking until the cauliflower is extremely tender and easy to mash.

8. Remove the lid from the pot and in a food blender, process the soup until lump free.

9. Stir in the mustard along with the Worcestershire sauce and cheese and cook until the cheese is melted.

10. Add the hot sauce (if required and to taste).

11. Stir in the chopped turkey bacon and garnish with onions.

12. Serve.

Nutrition per Serving

(Calories 240 | Total Fats 12g | Carbs: 19g | Protein 14g |Fiber: 5g)

Cheese and Broccoli Egg Muffins

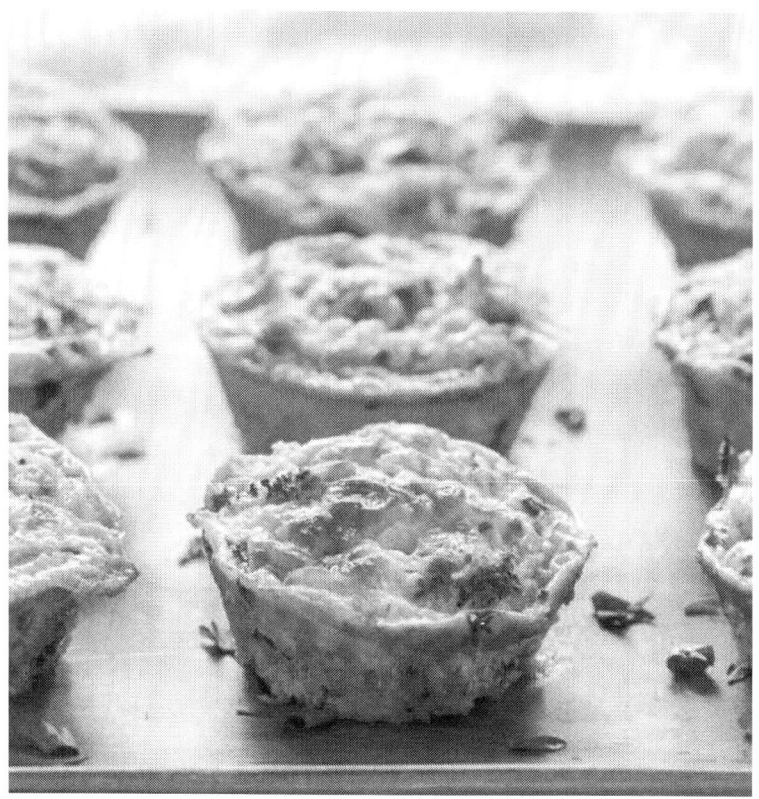

Scrumptious egg muffins are perfect for breakfast, brunch or a light lunch.

Servings: 4

Total Time: 50mins

Ingredients:

- 4 cups broccoli florets
- 1 tsp virgin olive oil
- Salt and pepper
- Nonstick cooking spray
- 1 cup egg whites
- 4 large eggs
- ¼ cup Pecorino Romano cheese (grated)
- ¼ cup reduced-fat Cheddar cheese (shredded)

Directions:

1. Preheat the main oven to 350 degrees F.

2. Add the broccoli to a pan with a little water and steam for 5-7 minutes. Set to one side to cool.

3. When the broccoli is sufficiently steamed, break it into smaller pieces and drizzle over the olive oil. Season with salt and pepper and mix to combine.

4. Spray an 8-cup, muffin pan with nonstick spray and divide the mixture evenly between the cups.

5. In a mixing bowl, beat the egg whites together with the eggs, and grated Pecorino cheese. Season.

6. Pour the mixture over the broccoli in the cups, to around three-quarters full.

7. Scatter with shredded Cheddar cheese and bake in the oven for 20 minutes, until the eggs set and the cheese bubbles.

8. Serve.

Nutrition per Serving

Cals 167 | Carbs 5g | Fat 8.5g |Fiber 2.5g | Protein 18g

Country Cajun Soup

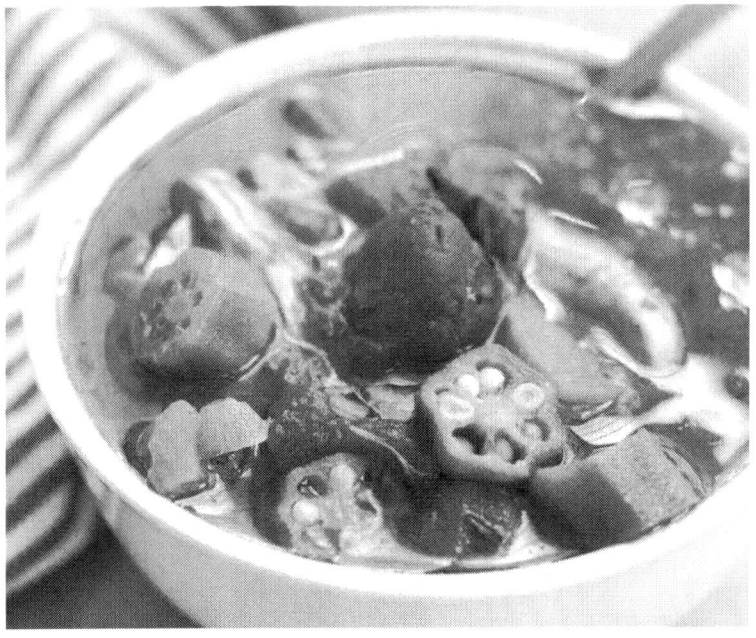

At only 93 calories per serving you can afford to keep coming back for more. This make-ahead soup is ideal for when you need to cater for a crowd.

Servings: 7

Total Time: 6hours 20mins

Ingredients:

- 1 tsp virgin olive oil
- ½ medium onion (peeled, chopped)
- ½ green bell pepper (chopped)
- 1 stalk celery (chopped)
- 1 clove garlic (peeled, minced)
- 3 ounces chicken andouille (chopped)
- 4 ounces lean ham (cubed)
- ½ (28-ounce) can fire roasted diced tomatoes
- 1½ cups water
- 1½ cups chicken broth
- 1 tsp Cajun seasoning
- 8 ounces frozen corn kernels
- Sea salt and black pepper

Directions:

1. Over medium heat, in a frying pan, heat the olive oil.

2. Add the chopped onion along with the pepper and celery and cook, while continually stirring until the veggies are fork tender, this will take around 5-7 minutes.

3. Add the minced garlic and continue to cook while stirring for 1 minute.

4. Transfer the mixture to a slow cooker and add the andouille, ham, tomatoes, water, broth, Cajun seasoning, and corn. Stir to combine and season.

5. Cover and cook for approximately 4-6 hours, covered, and until the veggies are softened and tender.

6. Season as desired.

Nutrition per Serving

Cals 93 | Carbs 10.5g | Fat 2.5g |Fiber 2g | Protein 8g

Crab Salad

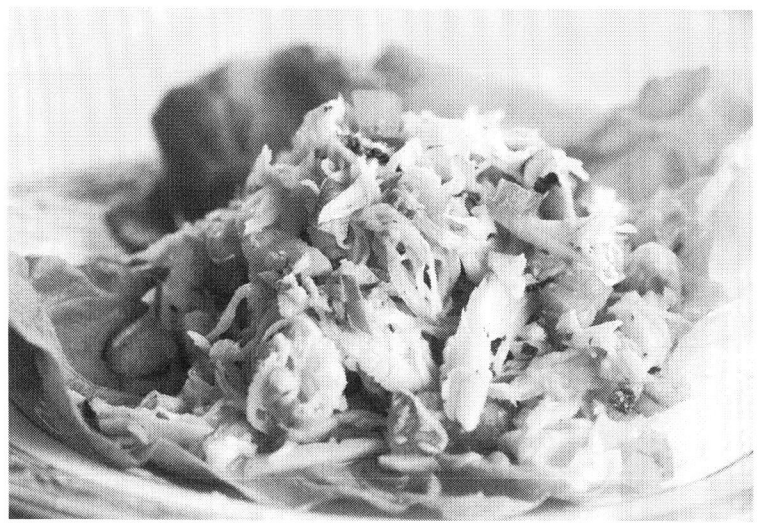

A light and refreshing crab salad is perfect for those get togethers with friend and at just over 100 calories per serving it's ideal for serving alongside a crisp and chilled white wine.

Servings: 4

Total Time: 15mins

Ingredients:

- 8 ounces lump crab meat (picked over)
- ¼ cup mayonnaise
- 2 tsp lemon zest (finely grated)
- 2 tsp freshly squeezed lemon juice
- 1 celery stalk (finely diced)
- 1 spring onion (finely chopped)
- 1 tsp Old Bay seasoning
- Dash Worcestershire sauce
- ½ tsp hot sauce

Directions:

1. In a bowl, combine all of the ingredients (crab meat, mayo, zest, juice, celery, onion, seasoning, Worcestershire and hot sauce and gently incorporate.

2. Transfer to the fridge to chill.

3. Serve.

Nutrition per Serving

Cals 110 | Carbs 5g | Fat 5g |Fiber 2g | Protein 11g

Garlic Pizza Bread

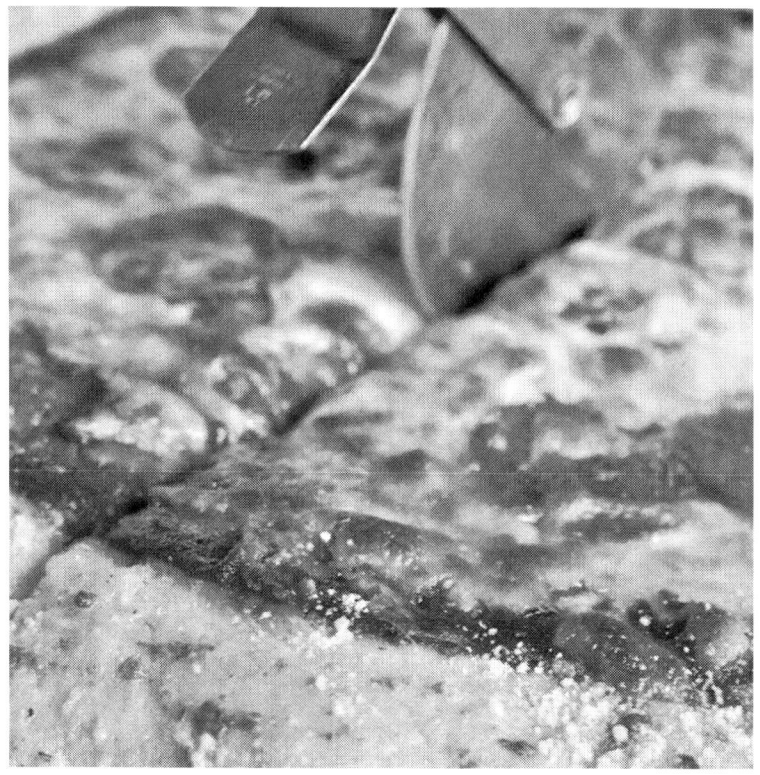

A delicious light bite to serve with drinks or a salad. Lots of flavor and super cheesy and at only 295 calories per serving you can enjoy this nibble guilt-free.

Servings: 4

Total Time: 25mins

Ingredients:

- 2 tbsp virgin olive oil
- 2 tsp garlic (peeled, minced)
- 2 (10") whole wheat pizza crusts
- 1 cup part-skimmed ricotta
- 2 tbsp Parmesan cheese (freshly grated)
- ¼ cup flat leaf parsley (chopped)
- 2 tsp pine nuts (toasted)
- Freshly squeezed black pepper

Directions:

1. Preheat the grill to moderate to high heat.

2. In a bowl, combine 1 tbsp of oil with the garlic.

3. Brush the pizza crusts on one side only with half of the garlic infused oil and place oil side facing down on the preheated grill and grill for 2 minutes, until the bottom of the crusts is golden.

4. Flip the pizza crusts over and brush with the remaining garlic-infused oil.

5. Scatter the top of the crusts with the cheeses and grill until golden, for 2 minutes.

6. Remove from the grill and sprinkle with chopped parsley, pine nuts, and black pepper.

7. Drizzle with oil, slice and serve.

Nutrition per Serving

Cals 295 | Carbs 28g | Fat 16.5g | Fiber 8.5g | Protein 12g

Hawaiian Grilled Cheese and Bacon Sandwich

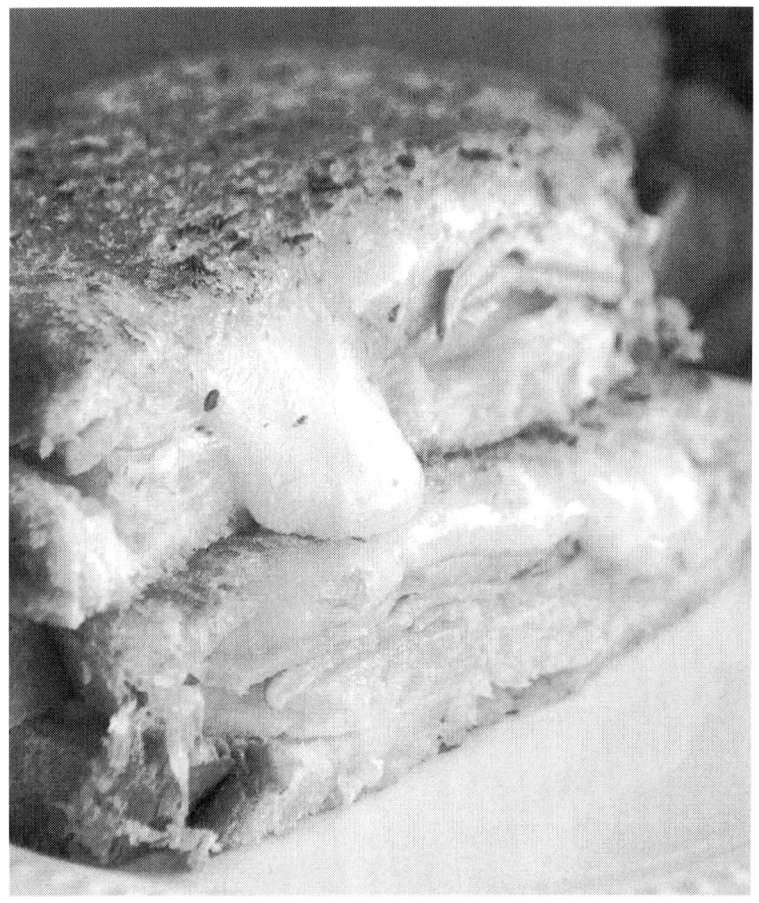

The perfect pairing; grilled cheese and pineapple with the added saltiness of bacon. Simply delicious and at only 160 calories a sure-fire weight watching winner.

Servings: 1

Total Time: 15mins

Ingredients:

- 1 tsp butter
- 2 slices thinly sliced bread
- Parsley
- Oregano
- 1 ounce Monterey Jack cheese (shredded)
- 3 slices bacon
- 3 slices fresh pineapple (peeled)

Directions:

1. Butter one side of each of the slices of bread. Scatter with parsley and oregano.

2. On the side of the bread, not buttered, sprinkle the cheese, top with the bacon, pineapple and the second slice of bread, butter side facing upwards.

3. Add the sandwich to a pan and cook over low heat until golden, flip over and cook on the other side until the cheese melts and the bread is lightly toasted.

4. Serve with a salad.

Nutrition per Serving

Cals 160 | Carbs 17g | Fat 9g | Fiber 2g | Protein 5g

Mediterranean Salad with Pulled Pork

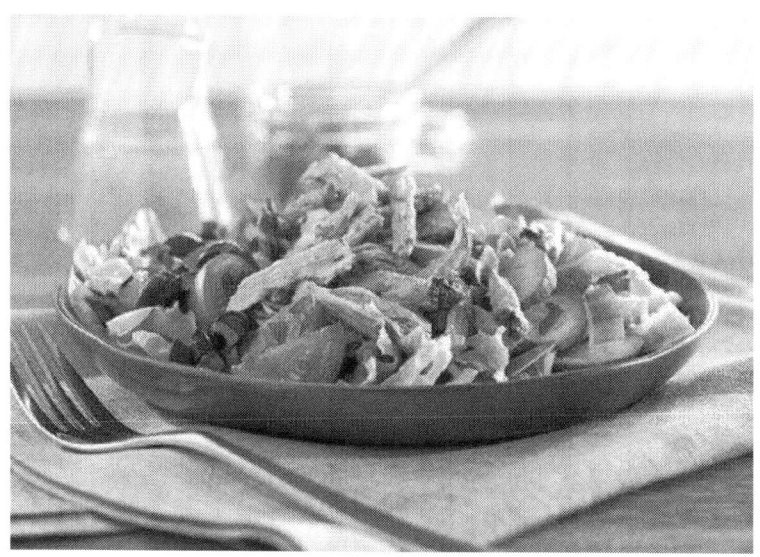

Pulled pork combines exceptionally well with a Mediterranean inspired salad. Lots of fresh veggies and lots of taste in every bite.

Servings: 4

Total Time: 7mins

Ingredients:

- 10 cups romaine lettuce (shredded)
- ¼ cup Italian salad dressing
- 1 pound pulled pork (cooked, shredded)
- 2 small tomatoes (cut into wedges)
- ½ cucumber (halved lengthwise, sliced)
- ½ red onion (peeled, cut into ¼ "dice)
- ½ cup feta cheese (crumbled)
- ½ cup kalamata olives (pitted, halved)

Directions:

1. In a large salad bowl, toss the lettuce with approximately half of the Italian dressing.

2. Arrange the tossed salad onto a serving platter and arrange the pulled pork on top.

3. Top with tomatoes, cucumber, onion, crumbled feta and olives.

4. Drizzle with the remaining Italian dressing and enjoy.

Nutrition per Serving

Cals 150 | Carbs 11g | Fat 10g | Fiber 4g | Protein 5g

Minestrone Soup

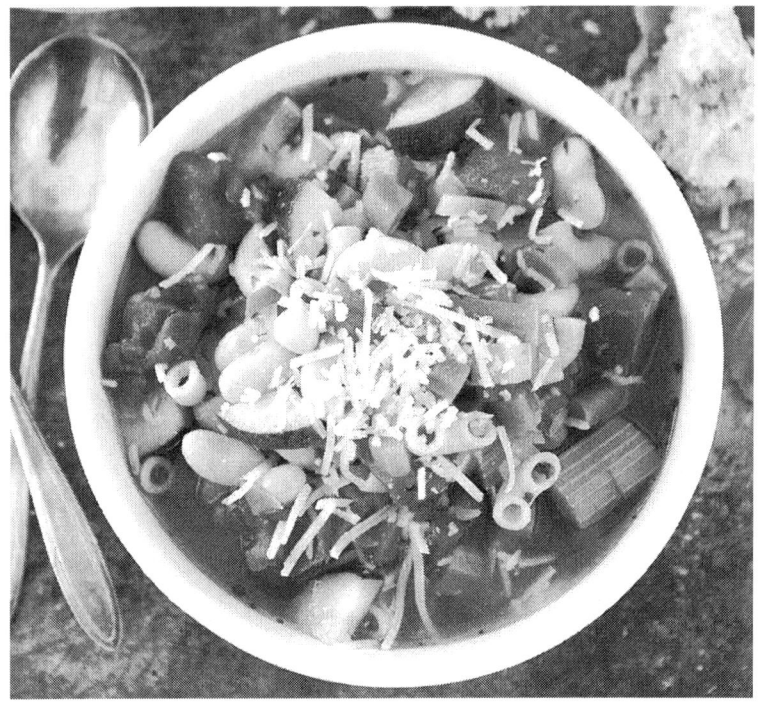

This Italian soup not only tastes good but it's packed full of veggies. So not only will you be enjoying a hearty and flavourful meal but you will be well on the way to your five-a-day.

Servings: 8

Total Time: 25mins

Ingredients:

- 2 cups small shell-shaped pasta
- 1 (15 ounce) can cannellini beans (drained, rinsed)
- 1 (32 ounce) container reduced-sodium chicken broth
- 2 tsp olive oil
- 1 cup carrots (diced)
- ½ cup celery (diced)
- ½ cup onions (chopped)
- 2 cloves garlic (peeled, minced)
- 1 (28 ounce) can petite diced tomatoes
- ½ tsp sea salt and black pepper
- 2 tbsp fresh basil (chopped)
- 1 fresh sprig rosemary
- ¼ cup fresh Italian parsley (chopped)
- 2 bay leaves
- 8 ounces zucchini (diced)
- 2 cups fresh spinach (chopped)
- Salt and pepper
- Parmesan cheese (to garnish, optional)*

Directions:

1. First, cook the pasta according to the package instructions, until al dente. Drain and set to one side.

2. In the food blender puree the cannellini beans along with the broth.

3. In a large frying pan over moderately high heat, heat the olive oil.

4. Add the carrots followed by the celery, onion, garlic and sauté until fragrant and for tender, for approximately 15 minutes.

5. Transfer the mixture to a pot along with the remaining chicken broth, diced tomatoes, bean puree, salt, and pepper. Add the basil, rosemary, parsley and bay leaves and cover. On low, cook for between 6-8 hours.

6. Approximately 40 minutes before the soup is cooked, add the zucchini followed by the spinach. Cover with a lid and cook for an additional half and hours.

7. Remove and discard the bay leaves and the sprig of rosemary. Season to taste.

8. Transfer the soup into 8 bowls along with ¼ cup of cooked pasta in each bowl.

9. Garnish with additional Parmesan if required.

*Remember to add the additional calories!

Nutrition per Serving

Cals 195 | Carbs 32g | Fat 3g |Fiber 8g | Protein 9g

Mushroom, Spinach, and Cheese Quiche

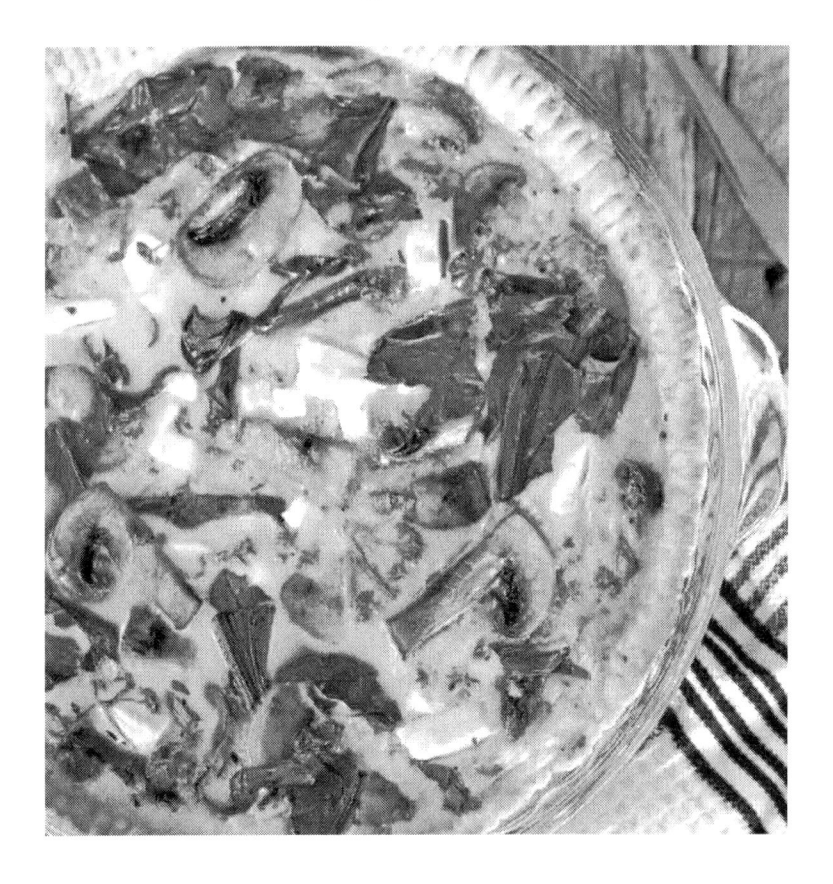

A tasty crustless quiche that is perfect to share. This meal is packed full of flavor, vitamins, and minerals thanks to the baby spinach. Healthy and wholesome, what more can you ask for?

Servings: 6

Total Time: 1hour 5mins

Ingredients:

- Butter (for greasing)
- 6 ounces baby spinach
- 2 cups mushrooms (coarsely chopped)
- 1 clove garlic (peeled, minced)
- Salt and black pepper
- 3 large eggs
- 1 cup half and half
- 1 cup Gruyere cheese (shredded)

Directions:

1. Preheat the main oven to 375 degrees F. Lightly butter a 9" pie plate and set to one side.

2. Add the spinach to a large frying pan and cook over moderate heat until wilted, this will take around 3 minutes.

3. Remove from the heat and spoon the mixture into a strainer set over a bowl. Set aside to cool.

4. Using the back of a spoon, firmly press and squeeze the spinach to expel as much moisture as possible. Place the spinach on a chopping board and roughly chop. Place the chopped spinach between two sheets of kitchen paper and press to expel moisture. Set to one side.

5. Using the same pan that you cooked the spinach in, over moderate heat, heat the oil.

6. Add the mushrooms and while stirring, cook until fork tender, for 5 minutes.

7. Add the garlic and cook for another 60 seconds.

8. Add the spinach and while stirring cook for 2 minutes, to ensure any moisture remaining has completely evaporated.

9. Remove the pan from the heat and season with salt and pepper.

10. In a bowl, whisk the eggs, add the half and half and stir to combine.

11. Spoon the spinach mixture into the prepared dish, scatter with shredded cheese and pour in the egg-half and half mixture.

12. Bake in the preheated oven for 30-35 minutes, until puffed, set and golden.

13. Serve.

Nutrition per Serving

Cals 220 | Carbs 5g | Fat 18g |Fiber 1g | Protein 12g

Mains

Chinese Chicken and Broccoli Stir Fry

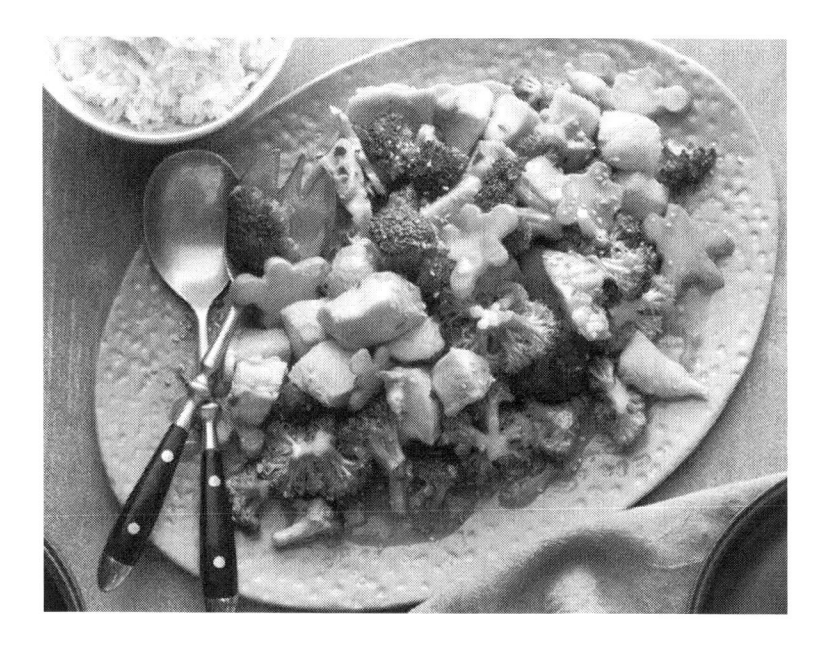

When the weekend comes around, and it's time for take-out, whip up this easy stir-fry instead!

Servings: 4

Total Time: 25mins

Ingredients:

- 3 tbsp light soy sauce
- 1 tbsp runny honey
- 2 tsp freshly squeezed lemon juice
- 2 tbsp sesame oil
- 1 tbsp cornstarch
- 2 tsp sesame seeds
- 1 tbsp virgin olive oil
- 1¼ pounds chicken breast filet (cut into bite-sized cubes)
- 1 onion (peeled, roughly chopped)
- 1 (1") ginger root (peeled, finely chopped)
- 2 cups broccoli florets
- ¼ tsp black pepper

Directions:

1. Whisk the soy sauce with the honey, fresh lemon juice, sesame oil and cornstarch and put mixture to one side.

2. Over moderate to low heat, in a large frying pan toast the sesame seeds for a couple of minutes, until they emit their fragrance. Put to one side.

3. Add the olive oil to the frying pan, turn to moderate heat and cook the chicken until golden.

4. Next add the chopped onions along with the ginger, broccoli florets, and pepper and sauté for 4 minutes.

5. Turn the heat down to moderate to low, add the soy sauce-cornstarch mixture and toss to combine evenly.

6. Continue cooking until the sauce is your preferred thickness, but for no longer than 5 minutes in total.

7. Garnish with the toasted sesame seeds and serve.

Nutrition per Serving

Cals 257 | Carbs 15g | Fat 18g | Fiber 5g | Protein 11g

Curried Cod with Pea Slaw

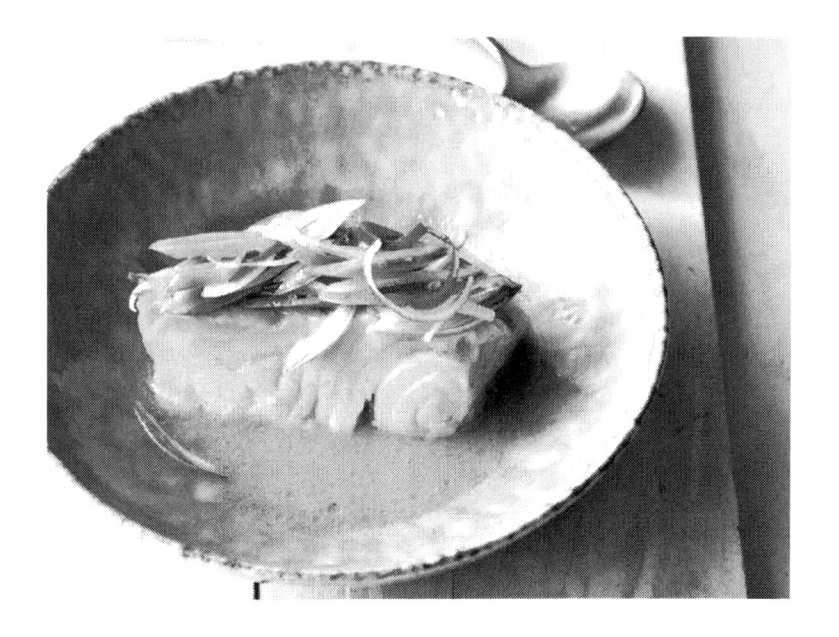

This recipe is proof positive that you don't have to sacrifice taste for calories. Coming in at just under 280 calories per servings it's the perfect choice for anyone watching their weight!

Servings: 4

Total Time: 30mins

Ingredients:

- 1 cup salt-free chicken stock
- ½ cup dry white wine
- 3 tbsp curry paste
- 4 cloves garlic (peeled, crushed)
- 1 bay leaf
- 1 (6 ounce) skinless cod fillets
- ⅔ cup sugar snap peas (thinly sliced across the diagonal)
- ½ cup yellow bell peppers (thinly sliced)
- ¼ cup shallots (thinly sliced)
- 1½ ounces tinned bamboo shoots (drained)
- 1 small Fresno chile (seeded, thinly sliced)
- 2 tbsp freshly squeezed lime juice
- 2 tbsp virgin olive oil (divided)
- ½ tsp kosher salt (divided)

Directions:

1. In a large pan, bring the chicken stock, wine, curry paste, crushed garlic and bay leaf to boil. Reduce the heat and add the cod. Cover with a lid and simmer for 7-10 minutes, until the fish flakes easily when using a fork. Remove the pan from the heat.

2. In a mixing bowl, combine the peas with the peppers, shallot, bamboo shoots, chile and fresh lime juice. Stir to incorporate.

3. Add 1 tbsp of olive oil and ¼ tsp of kosher salt and stir.

4. Take 4 bowls and add 1 cold fillet to each bowl. Sprinkle each fillet with salt and add approximately 3 tbsp of the fish poaching liquid to each of the 4 bowls.

5. Top each bowl with the pea-lime juice mixture and drizzle with the remaining oil.

6. Serve.

Nutrition per Serving

Cals 277 | Carbs 11g | Fat 10.1g |Fiber 2g | Protein 29g

Green Pesto Penne with Flaked Almonds

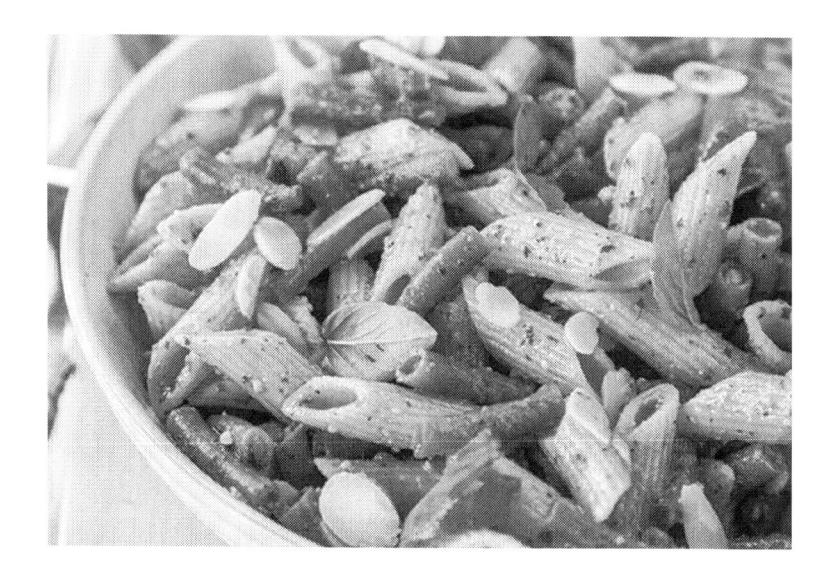

Combine texture and flavor in this easy to prepare pesto penne dish which is pot to plate in just half an hour.

Servings: 6

Total Time: 30mins

Ingredients:

- ½ tsp sea salt
- 4 ounces green beans (ends cut off, sliced into 1 ½ "long beans)
- 8 ounces whole grain penne
- 1 cup green pesto (any brand)
- ⅛ cup almonds (flaked)
- 8 large fresh basil leaves (roughly chopped)
- 4 tbsp virgin olive oil

Directions:

1. Over moderate to high heat, bring a pot of water to boil. When boiling, add the salt.

2. Add the green beans to the boiling salted water and cook for 5 minutes.

3. Transfer the cooked beans to an ice-water filled bowl. When the beans are sufficiently cool, drain and set to one side.

4. Using the same pot and boiling water, cook the penne according to the package instructions and until al dente. When the penne is cooked, drain and set to one side.

5. In a bowl, combine the penne with the green beans, green pesto, flaked almonds and chopped basil. Mix to incorporate.

6. Drizzle with oil and enjoy.

Nutrition per Serving

Cals 298 | Carbs 35g | Fat 14g |Fiber 3g | Protein 8g

Moroccan Chicken

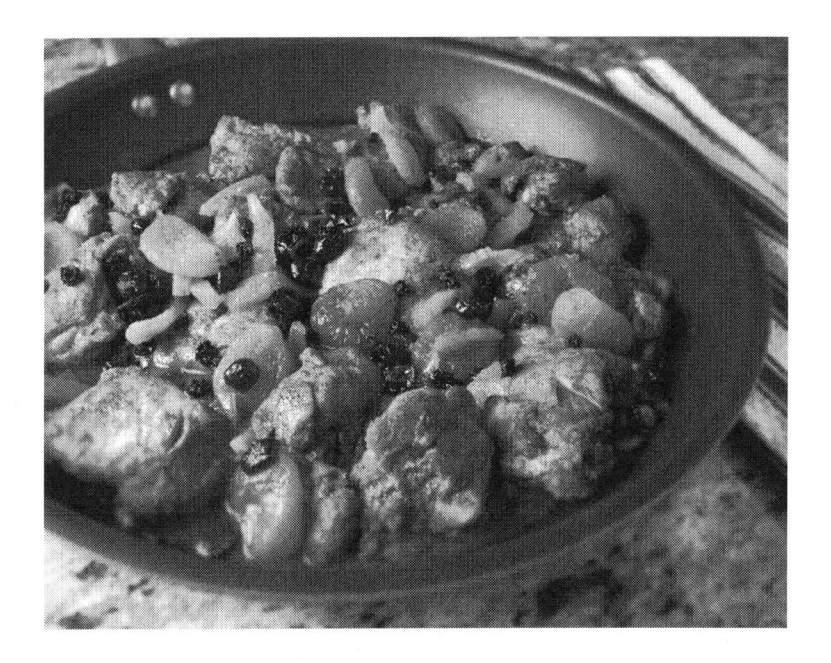

This African dish has lashings of flavor and texture but is low in fat, and calories.

Servings: 4

Total Time: 35mins

Ingredients:

- 4 (6 ounce) skinless chicken breasts
- 1 tsp ground cumin
- Black pepper
- 1 tbsp virgin olive oil
- 1 medium onion (peeled, finely sliced)
- 1 (14 ounce) can cherry tomatoes
- 1 cup water
- 2 tsp harissa paste
- 1 tbsp runny honey
- 2 medium zucchini (thickly sliced)
- 1 (14 ounce) can chickpeas (drained, rinsed)

Directions:

1. First season the breasts with cumin and black pepper.

2. Heat the oil in a large skillet and cook the chicken along with the onion for 4 minutes.

3. Flip the chicken oven and cook for an additional 3 minutes, while stirring the onions around the chicken breasts as they are cooking.

4. Tip the tomatoes in along with 1 cup of water into the pan and stir in the harissa followed by the honey, zucchini, and chickpeas.

5. Bring to a simmer and cook the chicken until tender for approximately 15 minutes.

6. Serve.

Nutrition per Serving

Cals 293 | Carbs 22g | Fat 6g |Fiber 4g | Protein 36g

Pan Seared Tuna with Ginger

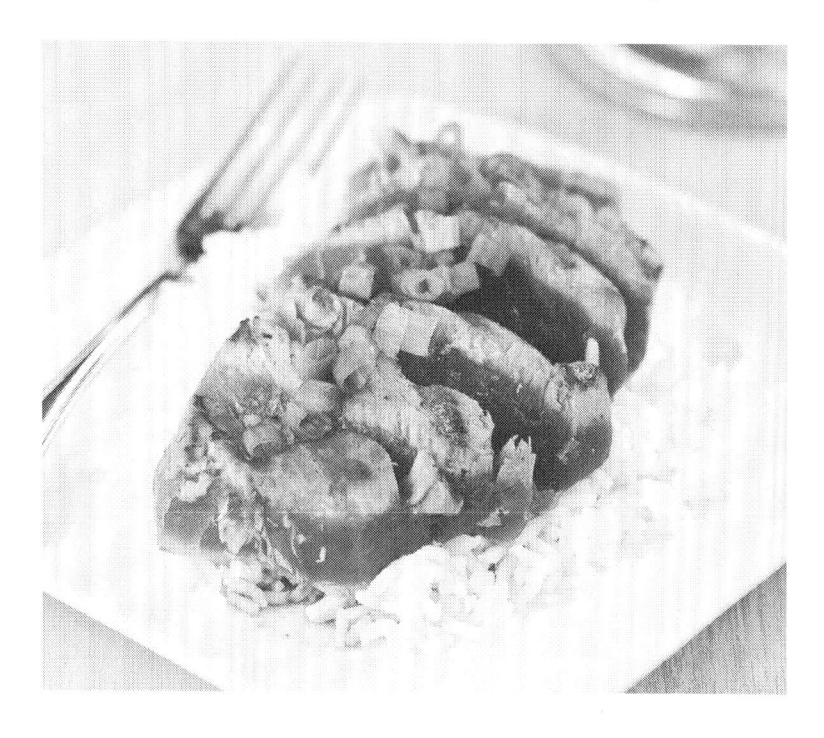

An Asian inspired main course that is guaranteed to be a big hit with all the family.

Servings: 4

Total Time: 1hour 45mins

Ingredients:

- 1 tbsp sesame oil
- ⅓ cup low-salt soy sauce
- 2 garlic cloves (peeled, minced)
- Freshly squeezed juice of 1 lime
- 1 tsp fresh ginger (grated)
- 1 green onion (chopped)
- 4 (4 ounces) tuna steaks
- Green onions (sliced, for garnish)

Directions:

1. In a bowl, combine the sesame oil with the soy sauce, garlic, lime juice, ginger and onion and stir to make a marinade.

2. Add the fillets of tuna to the marinade, cover, and place in the fridge to chill for 90 minutes.

3. Spray a large frying pan with cooking spray and set over moderate to high heat.

4. Sear the tuna in the pan for 60-90 seconds, on each side; timings will depend on how rare you like them.

5. Remove the tuna from the pan and serve, garnished with green onions.

Nutrition per Serving

Cals 210 | Carbs 2g | Fat 5g |Fiber 0g | Protein 27g

Pork Chops Italian Style

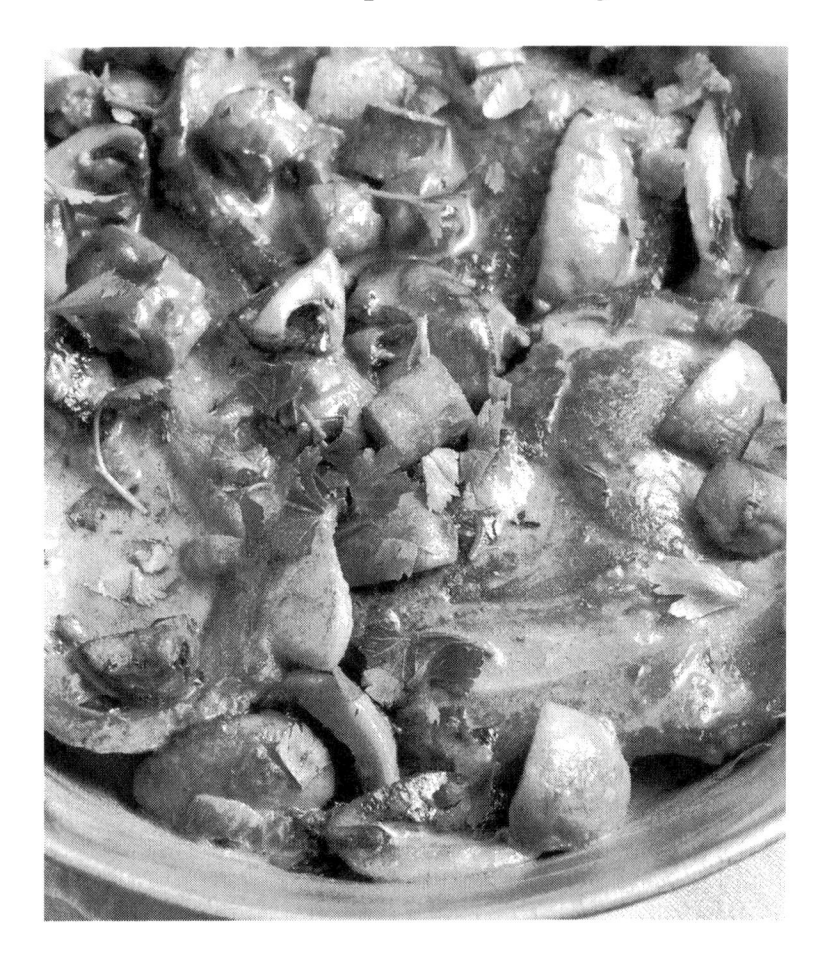

There are bound to be times when you crave red meat and these Italian style pork chops combined with mushrooms, wine and mozzarella are a delicious option.

Servings: 8

Total Time: 55mins

Ingredients:

- ¼ cup butter (divided)
- 8 ounces mushrooms (stemmed, sliced)
- ½ cup flour
- 8 thinly cut, boneless center pork chops
- 1 cup dry red wine
- ½ cup chicken stock
- Salt and black pepper
- ¾ cup mozzarella (shredded)
- 2 green onions (chopped)

Directions:

1. Melt 2 tbsp of butter in a large frying pan, add the mushrooms and sauté for 5 minutes until they begin to caramelize.

2. Remove the mushrooms from the pan and set to one side.

3. Lightly grease a 12x9" casserole dish.

4. Using the same pan, melt 1 tbsp of butter.

5. Pour the flour onto a plate and dredge the pork in the flour.

6. Add half of the chops to the pan and cook well, on each side.

7. Add the remaining 1 tbsp butter to the pan and brown the remaining pork chops

8. Transfer the cooked chops to the dish and scatter the mushrooms on top.

9. Pour the wine and chicken stock into the same pan you used to brown the chops, scraping the sides and bottom of the pan. Season with salt and black pepper.

10. Bring the liquid to a boil, reduce to simmer and on low cook for 10 minutes.

11. Preheat the main oven to 450 degrees F.

12. Pour the wine-chicken stock mixture over the pork chops and mushrooms in the casserole dish.

13. In a bowl, combine the shredded mozzarella with the green onions and scatter over the top of the meat.

14. Bake in the preheated oven for between 15-20 minutes, until the cheese melts.

Nutrition per Serving

Cals 150 | Carbs 11g | Fat 8g |Fiber 1g | Protein 3g

Rib-Eye Steak Caprese

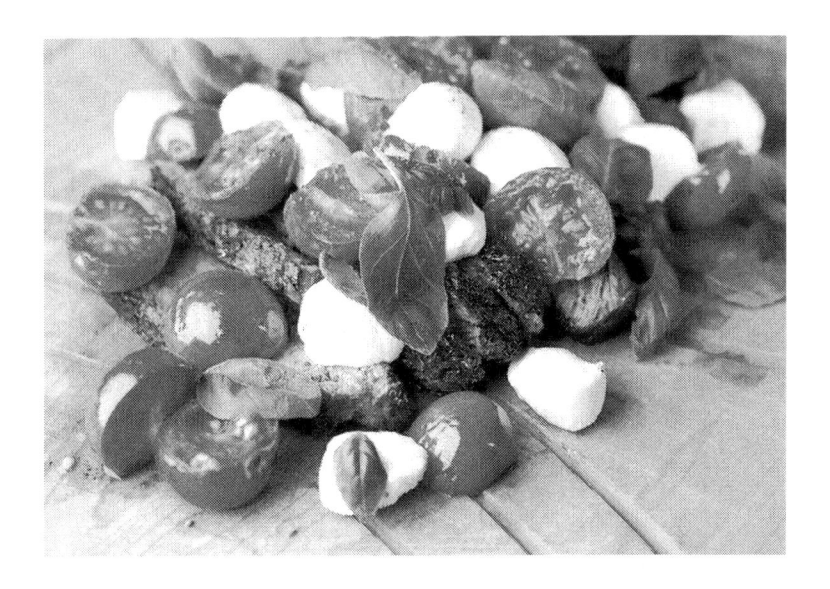

Tender and juicy steak grilled to perfection served with pan-fried tomatoes and mozzarella cheese is delicious and satisfying.

Servings: 4

Total Time: 25mins

Ingredients:

- 1 pound boneless rib-eye steak
- 2 tbsp olive oil
- 1 pint cherry tomatoes
- 1 cup mozzarella balls (room temperature)
- Basil leaves
- Sea salt and freshly ground black pepper

Directions:

1. Grill the rib-eye to your preferred level of doneness, 8 minutes each side for medium to well or 4 minutes each side for rare. Cover with aluminum foil and set the steak to one side to rest for 5 minutes before thinly slicing.

2. In the meantime, while the steak cooks heat the olive oil in a frying pan over moderately high heat. Add the cherry tomatoes and sauté for 4-5 minutes, until slightly softened.

3. Arrange the slices of grilled steak on a serving platter. Scatter the pan-fried tomatoes on top along with the balls or mozzarella.

4. Garnish with basil leaves and season.

Nutrition per Serving

Cals 180 | Carbs 5g | Fat 14g | Fiber 1g | Protein 8g

Rosemary Chicken with Oven-Roasted Veggie

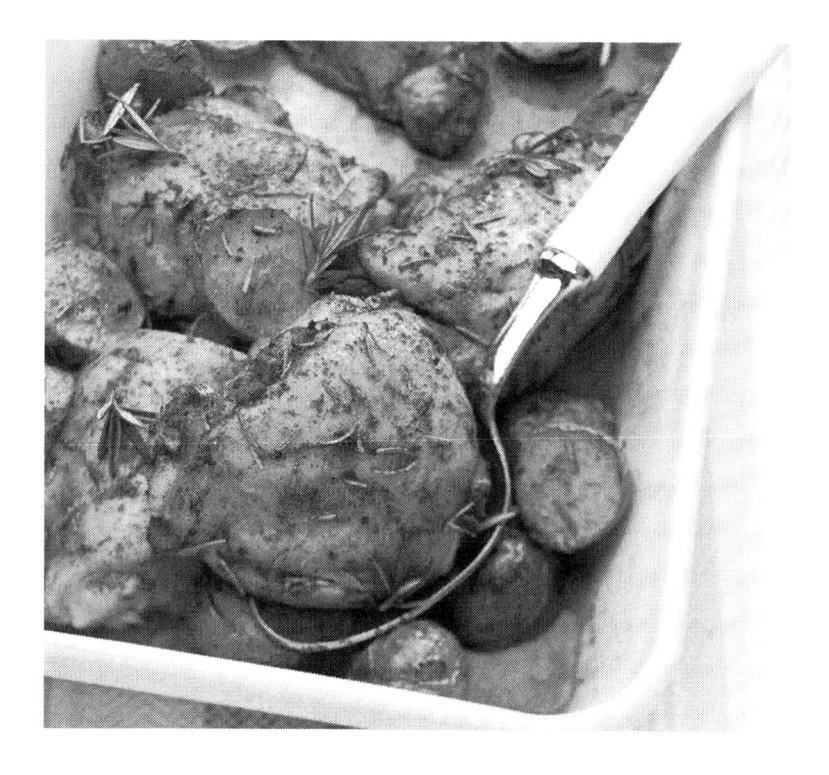

A low-calorie meal that all the family can enjoy is a real time-saver. This meal is an ideal one-pot chicken dish to enjoy with baby potatoes.

Servings: 4

Total Time: 40mins

Ingredients:

- 1 eggplant (cut into chunks)
- 2 zucchinis (sliced into half moons)
- 3 peppers (deseeded, coarsely chopped)
- 2 tsp rosemary (finely chopped, divided)
- 2 large cloves garlic (peeled, crushed, divided)
- 3 tbsp virgin olive oil (divided)
- Salt and pepper
- 4 boneless, skinless chicken breasts
- 8½ ounces cherry tomatoes (cut in half)
- 4 sprigs rosemary

Directions:

1. Preheat the oven to 400 degrees F.

2. In a large pan toss the eggplant with the zucchini and peppers along with 1 tsp of chopped rosemary, half of the garlic, 2 tbsp of olive oil and a dash of salt and pepper. Arrange the veggies in a single layer on the pan and roast for 20 minutes.

3. In the meantime, combine the remaining chopped rosemary with the remaining garlic and oil.

4. Using a sharp kitchen knife, slash each breast of chicken 4-5 times, brush with the seasoned oil, season with salt and pepper and transfer to the fridge to chill for approximately 15 minutes.

5. Remove the veggies from the oven and stir in the cherry tomatoes.

6. Re-arrange the chicken breasts in the pan and place them in between the veggies.

7. Add a sprig of rosemary on top of each breast and return to the oven for 18-20 minutes, until the chicken juices run clear and the veggies are fork tender and beginning to caramelize.

8. Serve.

Nutrition per Serving

Cals 289 | Carbs 11g | Fat 11g |Fiber 5g | Protein 37g

Salmon Tacos with Lime Yogurt

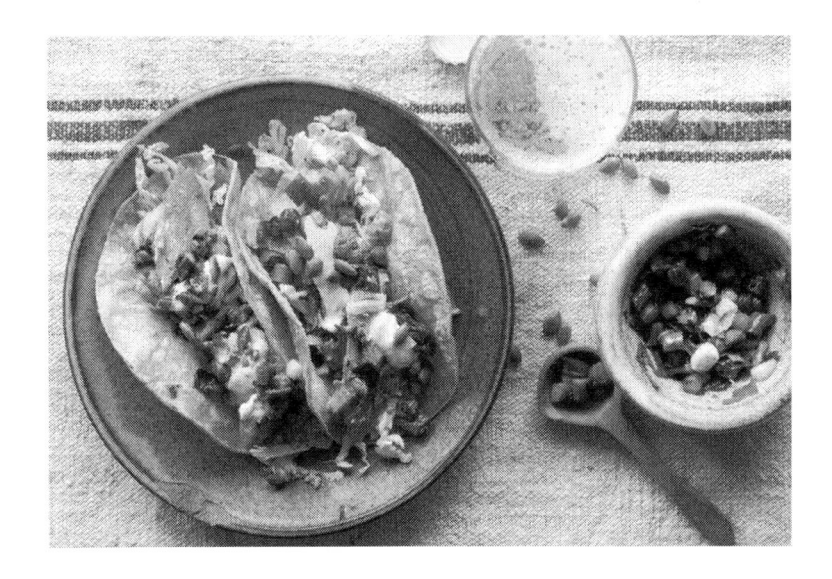

Meaty salmon combined with a citrus yogurt is a perfect light meal for summer.

Servings: 4

Total Time: 25mins

Ingredients:

- 1 tsp garlic salt
- 2 tbsp smoked paprika
- Pinch of sugar
- Salt and pepper
- 1 pound salmon fillet
- 1 cup fat-free yogurt
- 1 tbsp hot chili sauce
- Freshly squeezed juice of 1 lime

To serve:

- 8 small flour tortillas (warm)
- ¼ small green cabbage (finely shredded)
- Small bunch coriander (picked into sprigs)
- 3 pickled jalapeno chilies (finely sliced)
- Lime wedges (optional)
- Hot chili sauce (optional)

Directions:

1. In a bowl, combine the garlic salt with the smoked paprika, sugar, a pinch of salt and a dash of pepper. Rub the mix into the flesh of the salmon.

2. Heat the grill to high.

3. In a bowl, combine the yogurt, hot sauce and freshly squeezed lime juice with a little seasoning and put to one side.

4. Place the salmon fillets on an aluminum foil lined baking tray on the grill, skin side facing downwards until cooked through, for 6-8 minutes.

5. Remove the tray from the grill and peel off skin from the fillet.

6. Using a fork, flake the fillets into large chunks and serve with warm tortillas, prepared yogurt, shredded cabbage, coriander, sliced jalapenos, and lime wedges.

7. Add a dash of hot sauce to taste.

Nutrition per Serving

Cals 297 | Carbs 8g | Fat 15g |Fiber 5g | Protein 33g

Swordfish Burgers

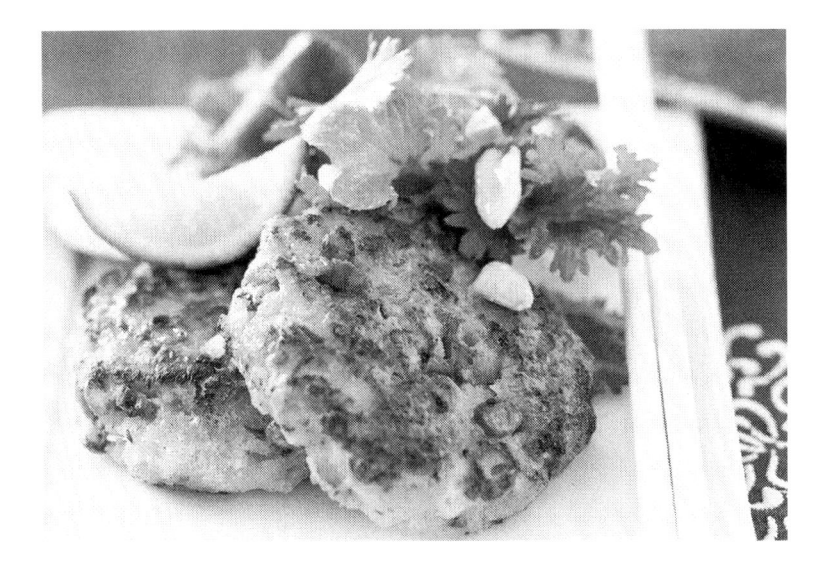

Swordfish is a really meaty fish and is perfect for burgers. Serve with a crisp green salad that will satisfy even the most difficult to please fussy eaters.

Servings: 4

Total Time: 35mins

Ingredients:

Dressing:

- Freshly squeezed juice of 1 lemon
- 8 tsp virgin olive oil
- Kosher salt and freshly ground black pepper

For the burgers:

- 4 (6 ounce) swordfish steaks (skinned, cut into chunks)
- 1 shallot
- 2 garlic cloves (peeled, chopped)
- 3 tbsp chives (chopped)
- Salt and black pepper
- ¼ cup breadcrumbs
- 2 tsp fresh lemon zest (grated)
- Nonstick cooking spray
- Iceberg lettuce (shredded)

Directions:

1. In a bowl, combine the lemon juice with the olive oil, and add a pinch of salt and a dash of pepper. Set the bowl aside.

2. Transfer 1 portion of the swordfish to a food blender.

3. Add the shallot followed by the chopped garlic and fresh chives. On the pulse setting, process to a thick paste. Transfer the mixture to a bowl.

4. Add the remaining portions of swordfish to the food processor and finely chop. Transfer the chopped swordfish to the bowl containing the paste and add a dash of salt and pepper, followed by the breadcrumbs and zest. Using clean hands, combine the mixture.

5. Form the mixture into 4 patties.

6. Lightly mist a frying pan with cooking spray and cook over medium to high heat, for approximately 4-5 minutes per side.

7. Serve with shredded lettuce and the lemon garlic dressing.

Nutrition per Serving

Cals 298 | Carbs 5g | Fat 16g |Fiber 1g | Protein 33g

Sweet Treats

Banana and Peanut Butter Cups

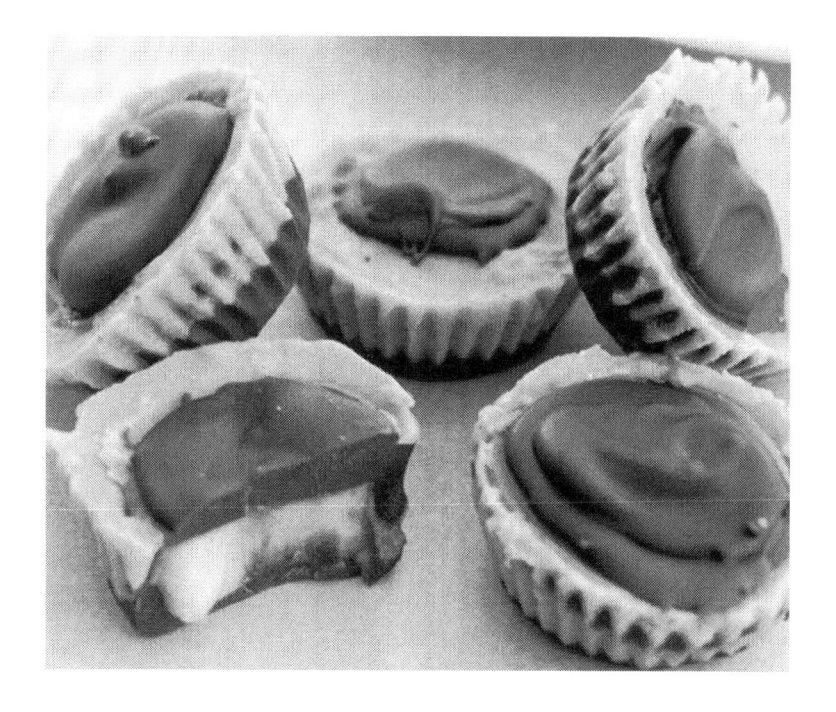

Super tasty pop in the mouth treats that you can keep in the freezer to satisfy those cravings for something sweet.

Servings: 16

Total Time: 2hours 10mins

Ingredients:

- ¾ cup dark choc chips
- ¼ cup organic smooth peanut butter
- 1 tbsp coconut oil (melted)
- 1 ripe banana (peeled, cut into 16 slices)

Directions:

1. Take a candy mold (minimum of 16, 1¼" holes).

2. Using a double boiler, melt the dark choc chips, set aside to cool a little.

3. Use a fork to whisk together the peanut butter and oil.

4. Drizzle 1 tsp of melted dark chocolate into 16 of the holes in the candy mold and arrange a slice of banana on top. Drizzle over 1 tsp of peanut butter followed by a final ½ tsp of melted chocolate.

5. Freeze for 1-2 hours before popping out and enjoying.

Nutrition per Serving

Cals 70 | Carbs 11g | Fat 4g | Fiber 1g | Protein 1g

Cheesecake Stuffed Strawberries

Sweet and juicy strawberries are stuffed with creamy vanilla, lemon cheesecake for an indulgent yet refreshing summer treat.

Servings: 12 (2 strawberries per serving)

Total Time: 3hours 10mins

Ingredients:

- 24 large, sweet strawberries (hulled)
- 8 ounces reduced-fat cream cheese (at room temperature)
- ½ ripe banana (peeled, mashed)
- 1 tsp fresh lemon juice
- 2 tbsp organic honey
- 2-3 drops calorie-free liquid sweetener
- 1 tsp vanilla essence
- 1 tbsp coconut sugar
- 1 tbsp almonds (crushed)
- Fresh mint leaves

Directions:

1. Pat dry the berries and slice a small piece off the point of each so that they can stand upright.

2. Add the cream cheese, banana, lemon juice, honey, sweetener, and vanilla essence in a bowl and beat until combined. Transfer the mixture to a piping bag (preferably with a star tip).

3. Pipe an equal amount of mixture into, and then on top of, each strawberry.

4. Sprinkle with coconut sugar and crushed almonds then garnish with fresh mint leaves. Chill for a few hours before enjoying.

Nutrition per Serving

Cals 100 | Carbs 9g | Fat 7g | Fiber 1g | Protein 2g

Chocolate Oatmeal Cookies

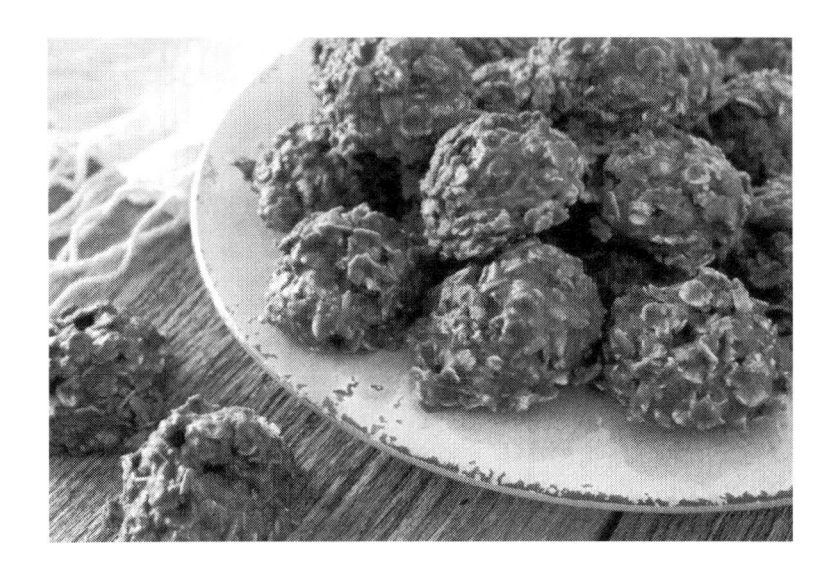

Chewy chocolate and oatmeal cookies naturally sweetened with maple syrup and coconut sugar are a yummy coffee-time treat.

Servings: 12

Total Time: 1hour

Ingredients:

- ¼ cup unsalted butter
- ¼ cup almond milk
- 3 tbsp cocoa powder
- 1 tbsp pure maple syrup
- 1 cup coconut sugar
- ½ tbsp almond essence
- 2 cups oats

Directions:

1. Cover a plate or cookie sheet with parchment.

2. Add the butter, milk, cocoa powder, maple syrup, coconut sugar, and almond essence in a saucepan over moderately high heat and bring to a boil.

3. While stirring, boil for 3-4 minutes then take off the heat.

4. Add the oats and stir until they are evenly coated with the mixture.

5. Drop spoonfuls of the mixture onto the parchment to make 12 equally-sized cookies.

6. Allow to cool and set up before enjoying.

Nutrition per Serving

Cals 205 | Carbs 35g | Fat 3g |Fiber 3g | Protein 5g

Cinnamon Spiced Apple Flautas

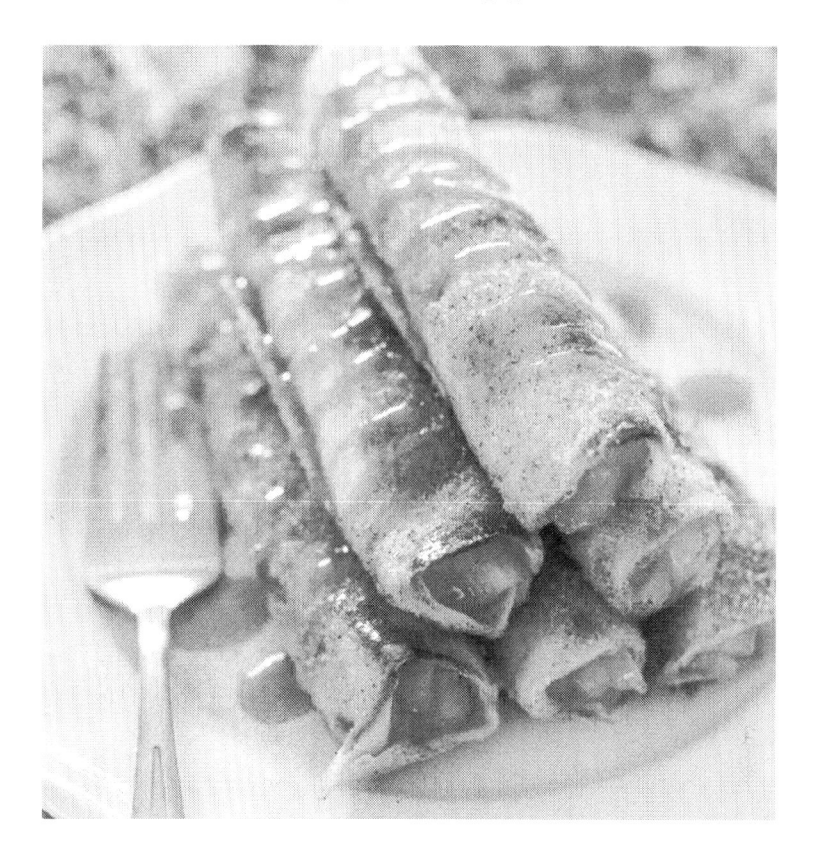

A delicious cinnamon-spiced apple filling is wrapped in whole wheat tortillas and baked until warm and fragrant.

Servings: 14

Total Time: 2hours 30mins

Ingredients:

- ½ tsp cinnamon
- 3 tbsp coconut sugar
- 4 Golden Delicious apples (peeled, cored, finely chopped)
- Pinch sea salt
- 1 tbsp cornstarch
- 2 tsp organic butter
- 14 small whole wheat tortillas
- Nonstick spray

Directions:

1. Add the cinnamon, coconut sugar, chopped apple, salt, cornstarch, and butter to a slow cooker. Stir well and cook for 2 hours on low heat.

2. Preheat the main oven to 350 degrees F and cover a cookie sheet with parchment.

3. Place 1 tbsp of the cooked apple mixture onto each tortilla and roll up as tight as possible.

4. Arrange the filled tortillas, seam-side-down, on the cookie sheet and spritz with nonstick spray.

5. Place in the oven and bake for just over 20 minutes until just crisp and golden.

6. Allow to cool a little before serving warm.

Nutrition per Serving

Cals 196 | Carbs 36g | Fat 4g |Fiber 3g | Protein 4g

Coconut Macaroons

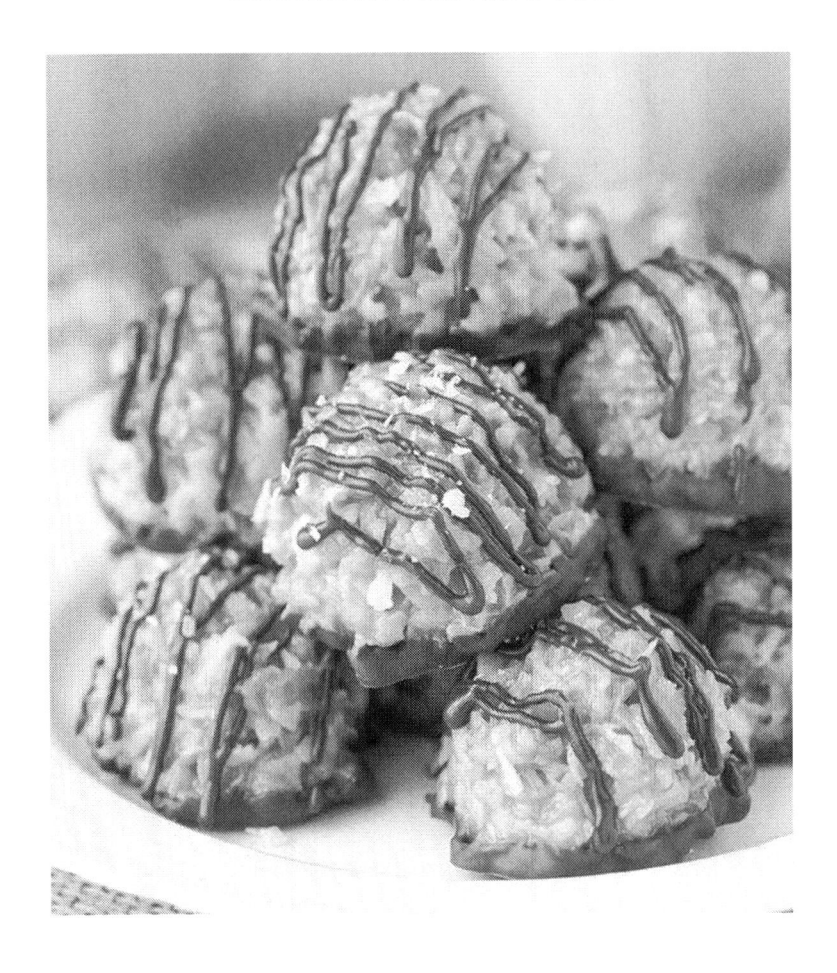

Chewy chocolate and oatmeal cookies naturally sweetened with maple syrup and coconut sugar are a yummy coffee-time treat.

Servings: 16

Total Time: 1 hour

Ingredients:

- ¼ cup virgin coconut oil
- ¾ cup organic honey
- 4 cups unsweetened shredded coconut
- 1 tbsp vanilla essence
- ⅔ cup cocoa powder (unsweetened)

Directions:

1. Cover a cookie sheet with parchment, set to one side.

2. Add the coconut oil and honey to a saucepan over low heat, Cook, while stirring, until melted and combined.

3. Add the shredded coconut, vanilla essence, and cocoa powder stirring to combine.

4. Drop spoonfuls of the mixture onto the parchment to form 16 equally-sized macaroons.

5. Freeze for half an hour until set before enjoying.

Nutrition per Serving

Cals 160 | Carbs 18g | Fat 11g |Fiber 3g | Protein 2g

Cookie Dough Balls

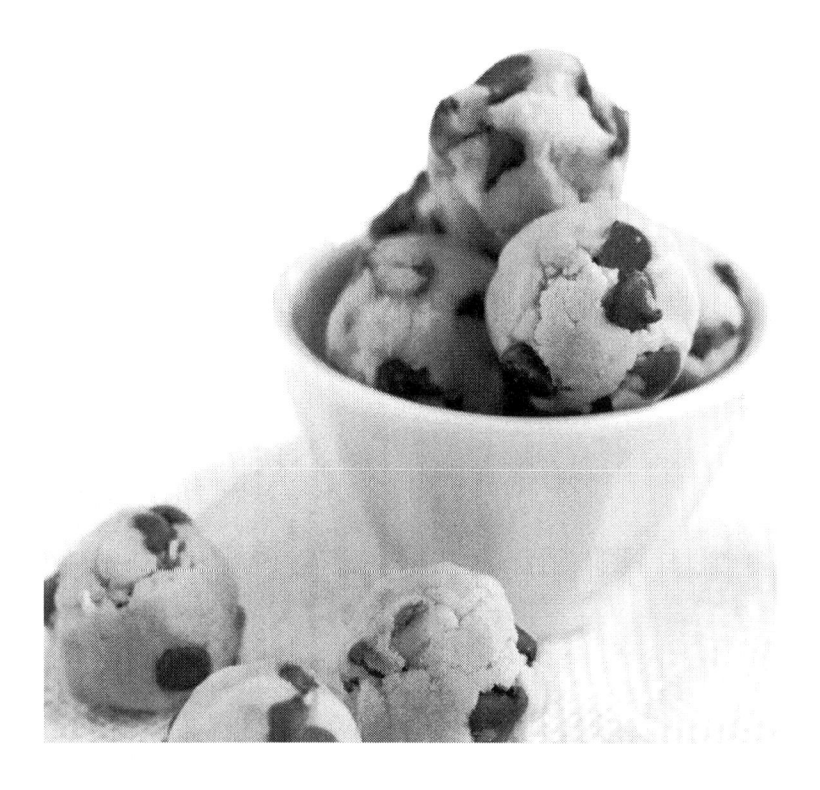

Who doesn't love licking the bowl when whipping up a batch of cookies?! These tasty balls have all the flavor of a fresh batch of choc chip cookie dough.

Servings: 12 (2 balls per serving)

Total Time: 45mins

Ingredients:

- ½ cup shredded unsweetened coconut
- 1 cup oat flour
- ¼ cup maple syrup
- ½ cup almond flour
- 1 tsp vanilla essence
- 1 cup smooth almond butter
- ¼ cup semisweet choc chips

Directions:

1. Cover a cookie sheet with parchment.

2. Add the shredded coconut, oat flour, maple syrup, almond flour, vanilla essence, and almond butter in a bowl and mix to combine. Add a little extra almond butter if the mixture is dry.

3. Fold in the choc chips.

4. Working with 1 tbsp of mixture at a time, roll the dough into smooth balls and place on the cookie sheet.

5. Chill until firm before enjoying.

Nutrition per Serving

Cals 255 | Carbs 19g | Fat 18g | Fiber 4g | Protein 7g

Gooey Peanut Butter Bars

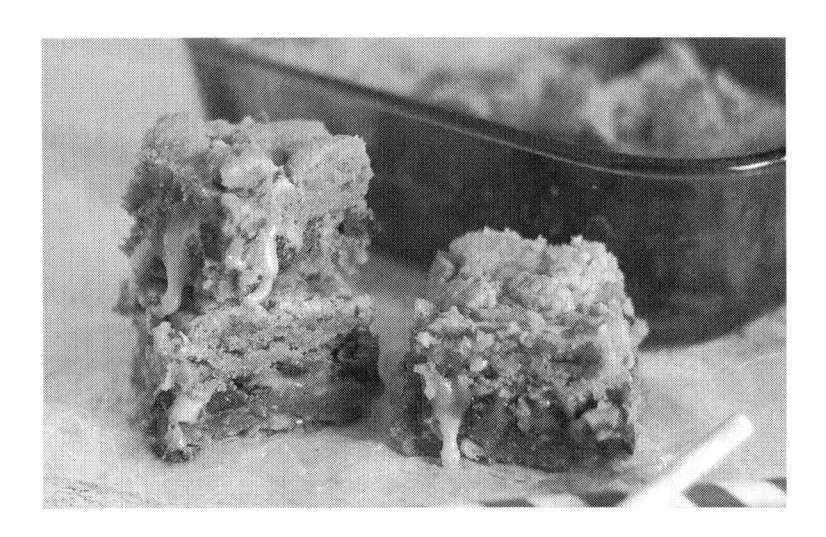

Oooey gooey bars topped with a sticky peanut butter frosting are a satisfying and scrumptious sweet snack or dessert.

Servings: 12

Total Time: 3hours 15mins

Ingredients:

Crust:

- 1 tbsp organic honey
- ¾ cup peanuts (finely ground)
- ¼ tsp kosher salt

- 1 tbsp virgin coconut oil (melted)
- 1 tbsp whole wheat pastry flour

Topping:

- ¼ cup coconut milk (from a carton, not a can)
- 1 cup organic smooth peanut butter
- 2 tbsp virgin coconut oil (melted)
- ¼ cup organic honey

Directions:

1. Line a square tin with parchment.

2. First, make the crust. Add the honey, peanuts, salt, coconut oil, and flour to a food processor, pulse until combined.

3. Press the mixture evenly into the base of the tin.

4. Next, make the topping. Add the milk, peanut butter, coconut oil, and honey to the food processor and blitz until smooth and combined. Spoon onto the crust.

5. Chill for a few hours, until firm before slicing into squares and enjoying.

Nutrition per Serving

Cals 235 | Carbs 14g | Fat 17g |Fiber 2g | Protein 9g

Lemon Berry Parfait

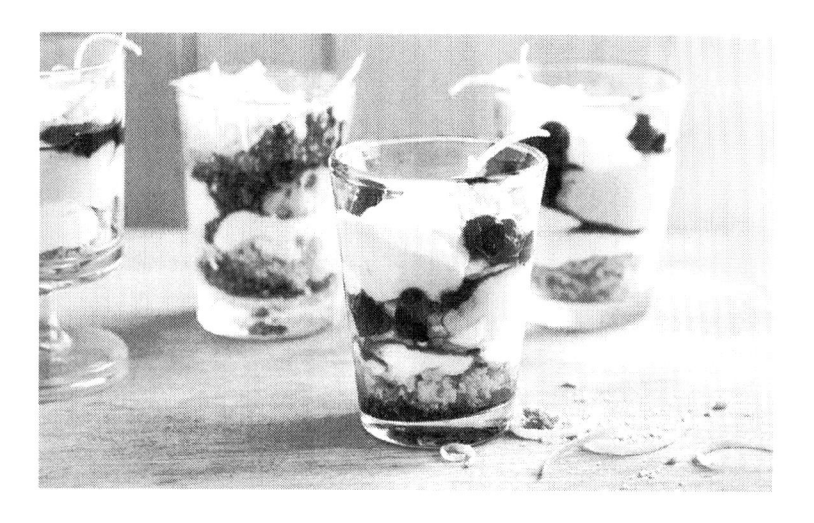

A tangy, sweet parfait with layers of fluffy lemon yogurt, sticky sweet date and pecan crumble, and fresh berries.

Servings: 6

Total Time: 10mins

Ingredients:

- Zest and juice of 1 medium lemon
- ½ cup reduced-fat cream cheese (at room temperature)
- 1 cup fat-free Greek yogurt
- 2 tbsp coconut sugar
- 2 large dates (pitted)
- ¼ cup pecans (chopped)
- 1 cup fresh berries

Directions:

1. Add the lemon zest and juice, cream cheese, yogurt, and sugar in a bowl. Beat until combined.

2. Add the dates and pecans to a food processor and blitz until crumbly.

3. In 6 serving glasses, layer equal amounts of the lemon yogurt mixture, followed by a little crumble and finally berries.

Nutrition per Serving

Cals 120 | Carbs 10g | Fat 7g | Fiber 1g | Protein 4g

Peachberry Sorbet

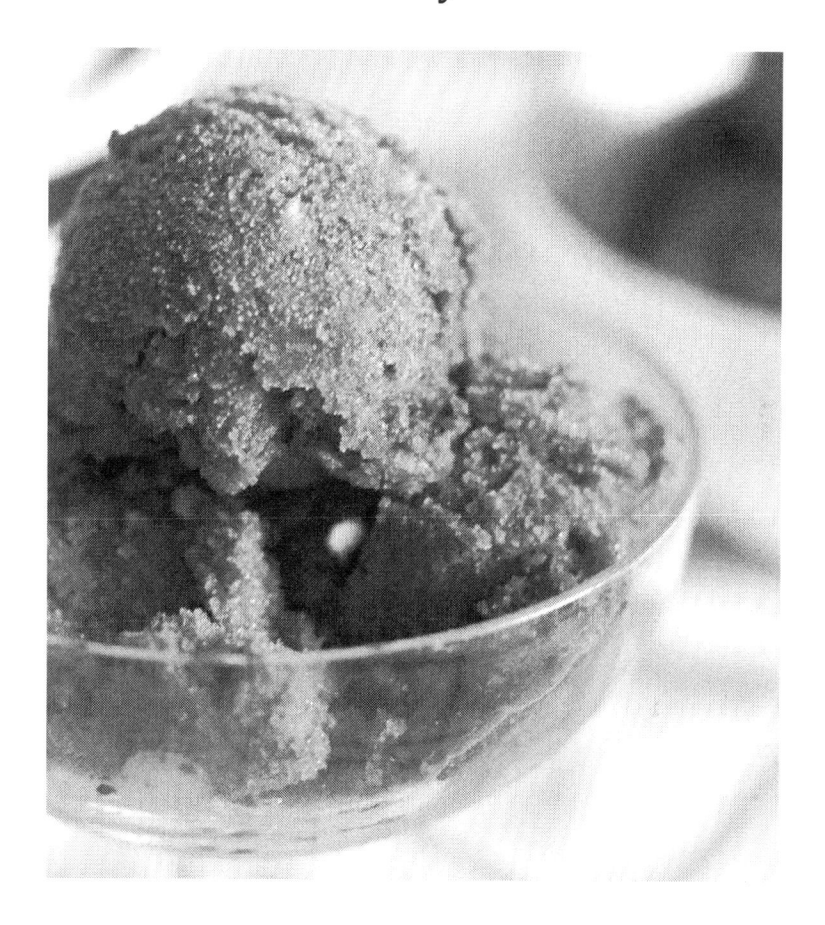

A refreshingly fruity sorbet perfect for cooling off on those hotter summer days.

Servings: 4

Total Time: 7hours 15mins

Ingredients:

- 1 tsp organic honey
- ½ tsp fresh lime juice
- 3 cups fresh peaches (peeled, stone, sliced)
- 1 cup fresh raspberries
- ¼ cup fresh orange juice
- ¼ cup canned no sugar added pineapple chunks + juice

Directions:

1. Add the honey, lime juice, and fruit to a bowl and stir well, transfer to a blender along with the fruit juices and pineapple chunks. Blitz until combined.

2. Pour the sorbet mixture into a resealable container and freeze for several hours until set.

Nutrition per Serving

Cals 85 | Carbs 21g | Fat 0.5g | Fiber 4g | Protein 2g

Ultimate Moist Brownies

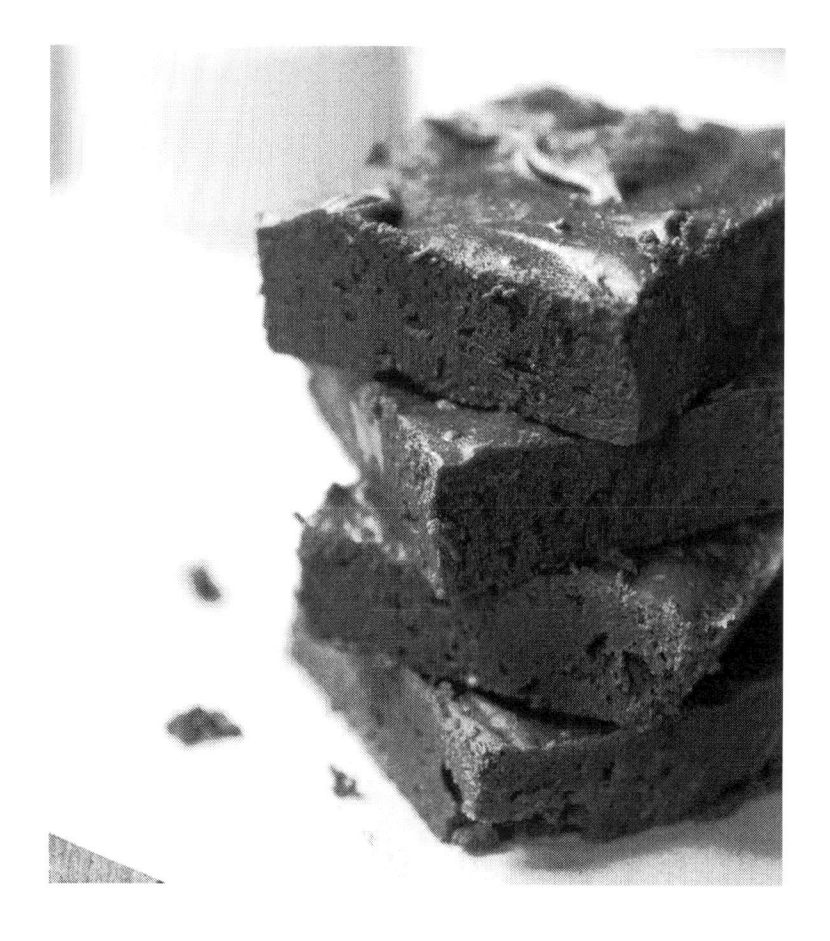

Moist, squishy brownies with all the texture but only a third of the calories. Why not serve warm with a dollop of your favorite yogurt for a yummy dessert?

Servings: 12

Total Time: 45mins

Ingredients:

- Nonstick spray
- 1½ cups canned black beans (drained, rinsed)
- ¼ cup blackstrap molasses
- ¼ cup applesauce (unsweetened)
- ⅓ cup cocoa powder (unsweetened)
- ¼ cup all-purpose flour
- ½ tsp kosher salt
- ½ tsp baking powder

Directions:

1. Preheat the main oven to 375 degrees F. Spritz an 8" square baking dish with nonstick spray.

2. Add the black beans to a blender, blitz until smooth and chunk-free. Transfer the black beans to a bowl along with the blackstrap molasses and applesauce. Mix well.

3. Add the cocoa powder, flour, salt, and baking powder to the black bean mixture and stir well until totally combined.

4. Transfer the brownie batter to the baking dish and place in the oven. Bake for just over half an hour.

5. Allow to cool to room temperature before slicing and serving.

Nutrition per Serving

Cals 120 | Carbs 24g | Fat 1g |Fiber 5g | Protein 6g

Smoothies

Bloat Buster

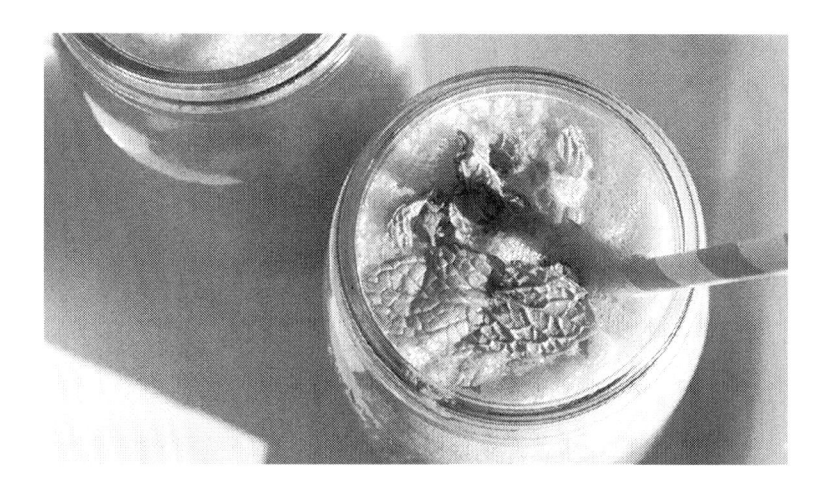

Bust uncomfortable bloat with this detoxifying smoothie made with zingy ginger, hydrating coconut water, and refreshing cucumber.

Servings: 1

Total Time: 5mins

Ingredients:

- 1 ripe, medium banana (peeled, chopped)
- ½ cup coconut water
- 1" chunk ginger (peeled, chopped)
- 1 cucumber (chopped)
- Ice

Directions:

1. Add the banana, coconut water, ginger, and cucumber to a blender along with a handful of ice. Blitz until combined.

2. Pour into a glass and enjoy.

Nutrition per Serving

Cals 170 | Carbs 44g | Fat 2g |Fiber 8g | Protein 5g

Cocoberry Smoothie

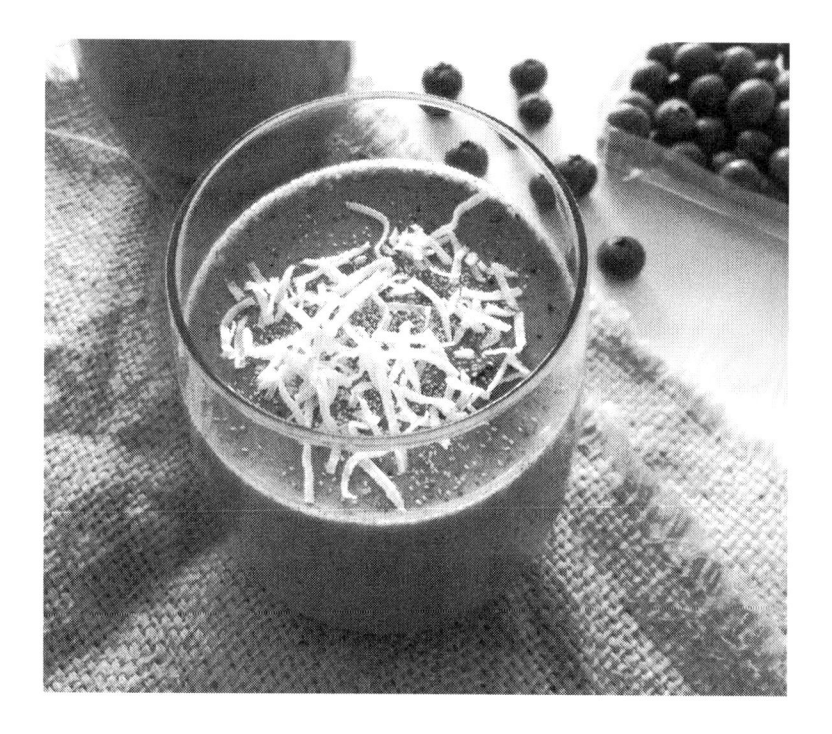

This protein-packed smoothie is a fantastic metabolism booster, the ideal drink to sip on when you're trying to shift those last few stubborn pounds.

Servings: 1

Total Time: 5mins

Ingredients:

- 1 (5.3 ounce) pot low-calorie coconut flavor yogurt
- 2 tbsp almonds
- 1 large banana (peeled, chopped, frozen)
- 1 cup fresh blueberries
- 1 cup almond milk
- ½ zero calorie sweetener
- 2 tbsp unsweetened coconut flakes

Directions:

1. Add the yogurt, almonds, banana, blueberries, milk, sweetener, and coconut flakes to a blender and blitz until combined.

2. Pour into a glass and enjoy.

Nutrition per Serving

Cals 280 | Carbs 38g | Fat 10g | Fiber 6g | Protein 10g

Fruity Green Tea Smoothie

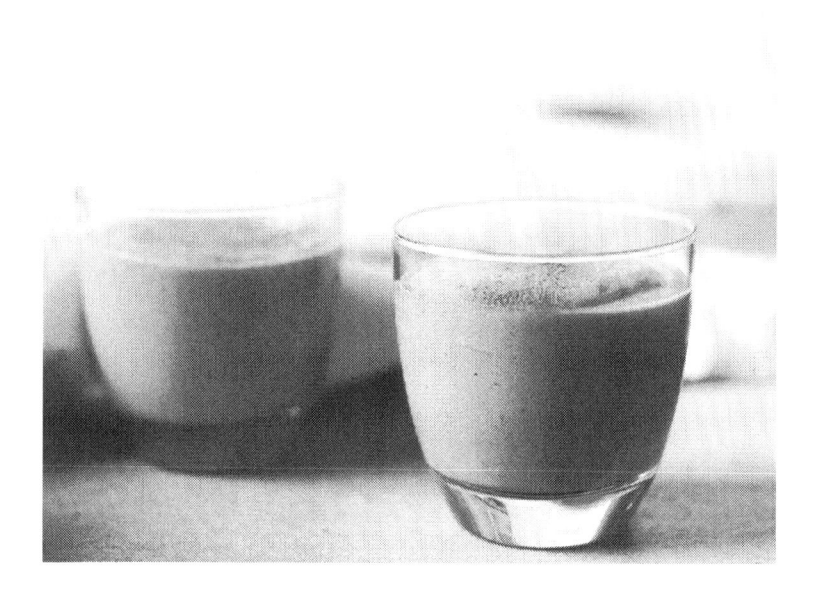

Green tea is full of healthy catechins and antioxidants, which help to fight cell damage and keep your body fighting fit. This fruity smoothie is a tasty way to get your daily dose of green tea.

Servings: 1

Total Time: 5mins

Ingredients:

- Pinch cayenne pepper
- ¼ tsp cinnamon
- ¾ cup extra-strong brewed green tea (cooled)
- ½ pear (peeled, cored, chopped)
- ¼ cup full-fat Greek yogurt
- 3 tsp organic honey
- ½ medium orange (peeled, chopped)
- ½ apple (peeled, cored, chopped)
- Ice

Directions:

1. Add the cayenne pepper, cinnamon, tea, pear, yogurt, honey, orange, and apple to a blender along with a handful of ice and blitz until combined.

2. Pour into a glass and enjoy.

Nutrition per Serving

Cals 210 | Carbs 42g | Fat 4g | Fiber 5g | Protein 7g

Key Lime Pie Smoothie

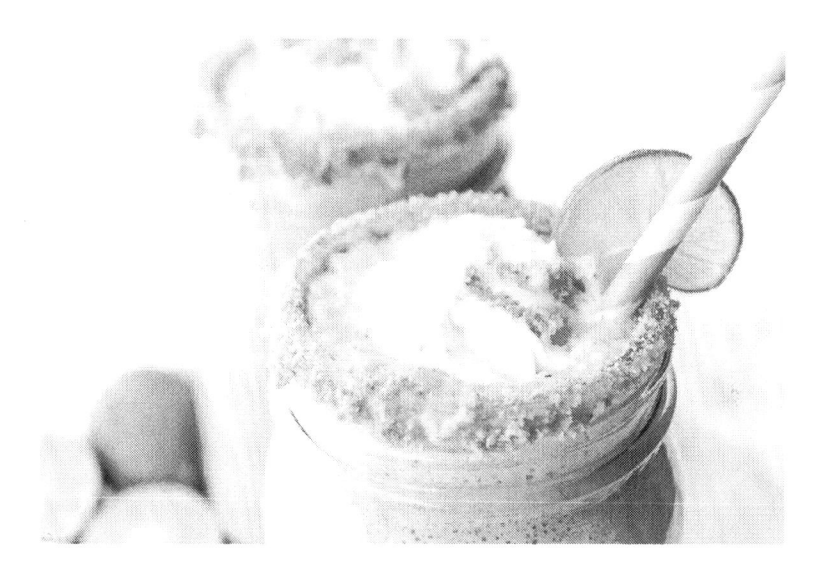

This tangy dessert-inspired smoothie is packed with protein making it an ideal pre or post-workout drink.

Servings: 1

Total Time: 5mins

Ingredients:

- 1 scoop vanilla flavored protein powder
- ½ cup reduced-fat cottage cheese
- ¾ cup water
- 1 tbsp Key lime juice
- Handful spinach leaves
- ½ tsp zero calorie sweetener
- Ice

Directions:

1. Add the protein powder, cottage cheese, water, lime juice, spinach, and sweetener in a blender along with a handful of ice and blitz until combined.

2. Pour into an ice-filled glass and enjoy.

Nutrition per Serving

Cals 210 | Carbs 17g | Fat 0g |Fiber 1g | Protein 42g

Mango Lassi

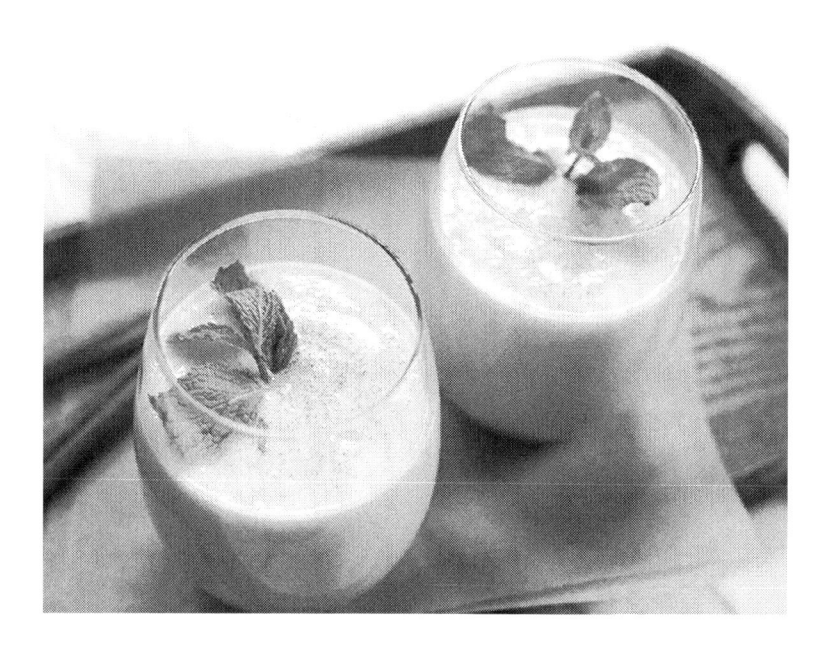

A thick and rich smoothie spiced with cardamom and cinnamon inspired by the popular Indian treat – lassi.

Servings: 2

Total Time: 5mins

Ingredients:

- Pinch ground cardamom
- 1½ cups fat-free plain yogurt
- 2 ripe mangoes (peeled, pitted, chopped)
- ¼ tsp cinnamon
- 1 tbsp organic honey
- ¼ cup coconut milk (from a carton, not a can)
- Ice

Directions:

1. Add the cardamom, yogurt, mango, cinnamon, honey, and milk to a blender along with a small handful of ice and blitz until combined.

2. Pour into glasses and enjoy.

Nutrition per Serving

Cals 210 | Carbs 38g | Fat 3g | Fiber 1g | Protein 10g

Mint Choc Chip Smoothie

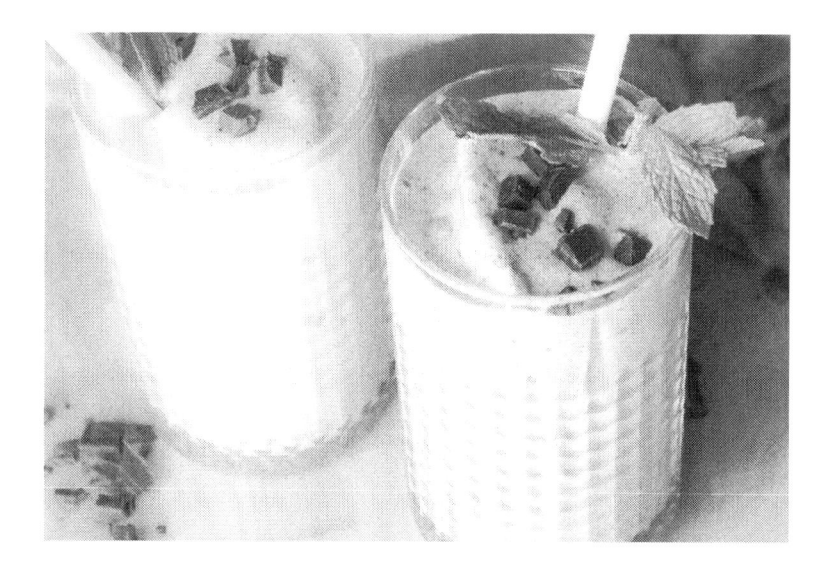

This yummy mint choc chip smoothie is made super satisfying and filling thanks to the addition of frozen bananas.

Servings: 4

Total Time: 5mins

Ingredients:

- Handful fresh mint
- 2½ ounces fresh spinach leaves
- 4 large bananas (peeled, chopped, frozen)
- 1 cup coconut milk (from a carton, not a can)
- 2 ounces dark chocolate (chopped)

Directions:

1. Add the mint, spinach, banana, and milk in a blender and blitz until combined.

2. Pour into glasses, sprinkle with dark chocolate and enjoy.

Nutrition per Serving

Cals 135 | Carbs 14g | Fat 8.75g |Fiber 2.5g | Protein 2g

Mocha Frappuccino Smoothie

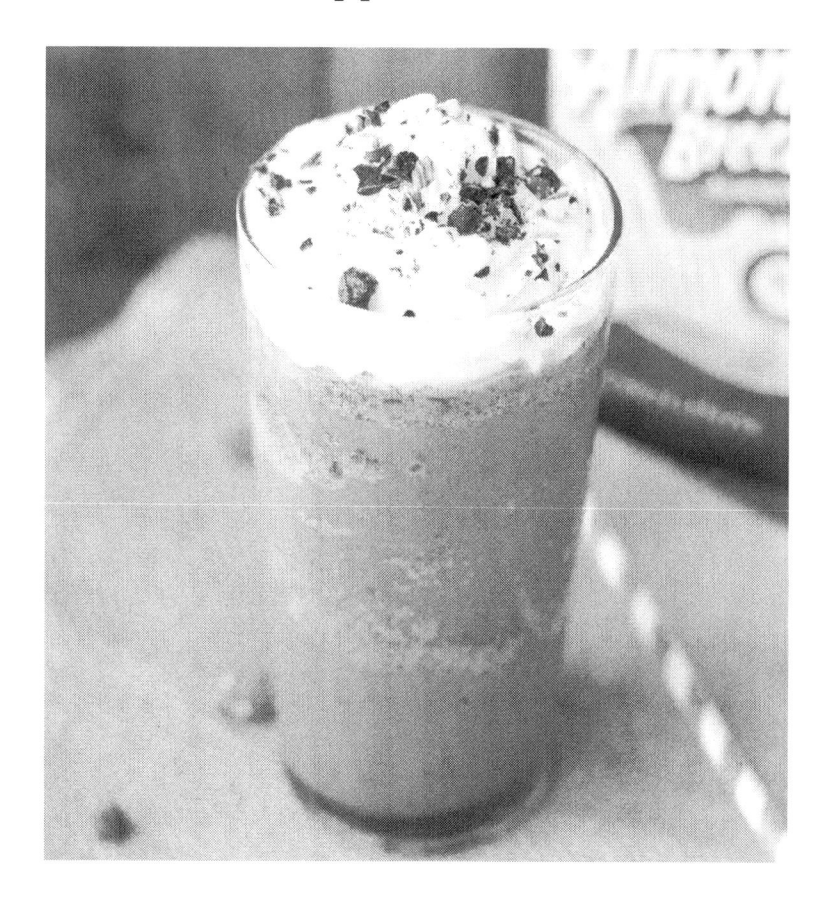

A healthy, protein-packed frappuccino with less than half the calories and fat of your favorite barista-style beverage.

Servings: 1

Total Time: 5mins

Ingredients:

- 1 scoop chocolate flavor protein powder
- ¼ cup extra-strong brewed coffee (cooled)
- 1 tbsp cocoa powder
- 1 tbsp flaxseed meal
- ¼ cup almond milk
- ½ cup ice

Directions:

1. Add the protein powder, coffee, cocoa powder, flaxseed meal, and milk in a blender along with the ice and blitz until combined.

2. Pour into a glass and enjoy.

Nutrition per Serving

Cals 120 | Carbs 7g | Fat 5g |Fiber 3g | Protein 12g

Pumpkin Pie Smoothie

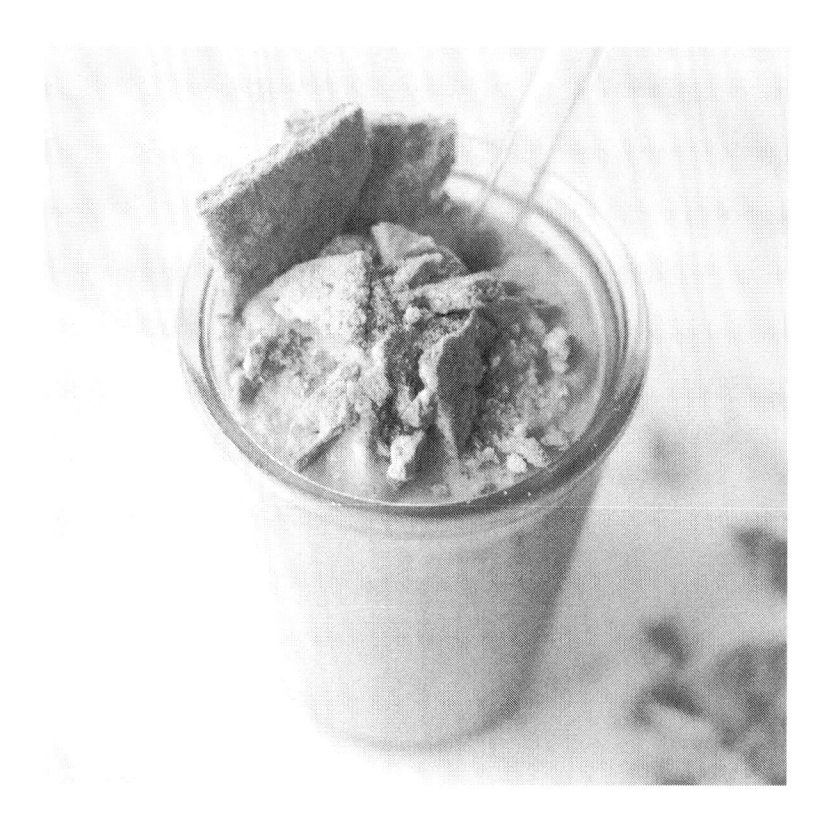

All the flavor of a deliciously spiced pumpkin pie in a glass! We can't think of a yummier way to start the morning or satisfy the mid-afternoon munchies.

Servings: 1

Total Time: 5mins

Ingredients:

- 1 large banana (peeled, chopped, frozen)
- ⅓ cup pureed pumpkin
- Pinch nutmeg
- 1 cup vanilla flavored almond milk
- ½ tsp cinnamon
- Ice

Directions:

1. Add the banana, pumpkin, nutmeg, almond milk, and cinnamon in a blender and blitz until combined.

2. Pour into an ice-filled glass and enjoy.

Nutrition per Serving

Cals 190 | Carbs 40g | Fat 3.5g |Fiber 9g | Protein 3g

Tropical Breeze Smoothie

With the tropical taste of mango, pineapple, and banana you'd never guess this yummy smoothie was chock full of vitamin-rich spinach!

Servings: 1

Total Time: 5mins

Ingredients:

- ¼ cup fresh mango (peeled, pitted, chopped)
- 1 handful spinach leaves
- 1 cup almond milk
- ¼ cup fresh pineapple (peeled, chopped)
- 1 tbsp chia seeds
- 1 tbsp flax meal
- 1 scoop vanilla flavor protein powder
- ½ medium banana (peeled, chopped)
- Ice

Directions:

1. Add the mango, spinach, milk, pineapple, chia seeds, flax meal, protein powder, and banana to a blender along with a small handful of ice and blitz until combined.

2. Pour into a glass and enjoy.

Nutrition per Serving

Cals 230 | Carbs 9g | Fat 8g |Fiber 9g | Protein 19g

Vanilla Cherry Smoothie

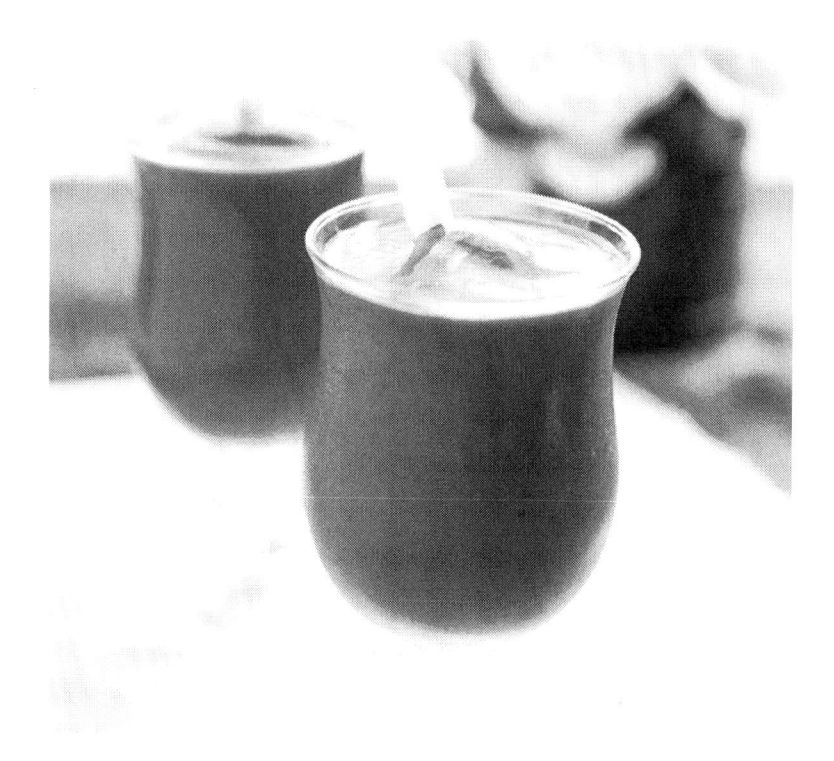

This delicious smoothie flavored with sweet cherries and creamy vanilla yogurt is guaranteed to be loved by all.

Servings: 1

Total Time: 5mins

Ingredients:

- ½ tsp vanilla essence
- ½ cup full-fat vanilla flavor Greek yogurt
- 1 cup frozen pitted cherries
- 2 tsp zero-calorie sweetener

Directions:

1. Add the vanilla essence, yogurt, cherries, and sweetener in a blender and blitz until combined.

2. Pour into a glass and enjoy.

Nutrition per Serving

Cals 120 | Carbs 25g | Fat 0.5g |Fiber 2g | Protein 11g

Author's Afterthoughts

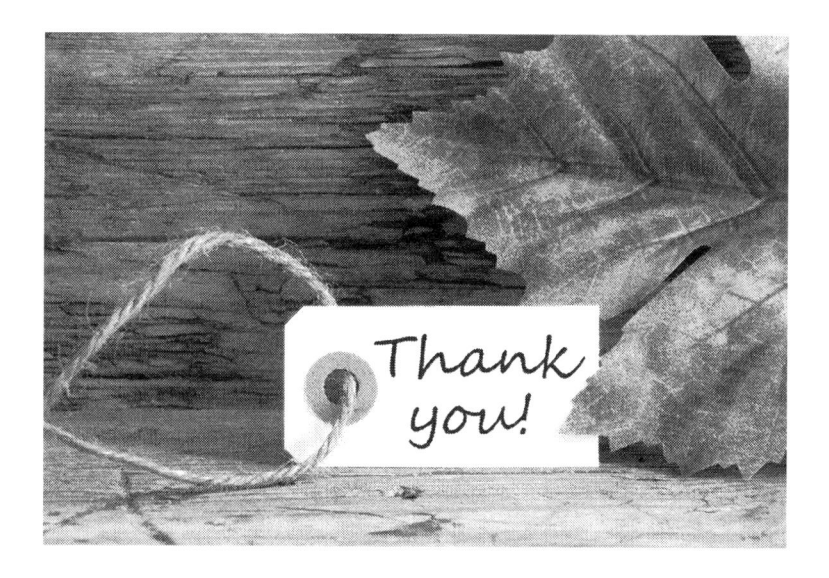

Thanks ever so much to each of my cherished readers for investing the time to read this book!

I know you could have picked from many other books but you chose this one. So a big thanks for downloading this book and reading all the way to the end.

If you enjoyed this book or received value from it, I'd like to ask you for a favor. Please take a few minutes to post an honest and heartfelt review on Amazon.com. Your support does make a difference and helps to benefit other people.

Thanks!

Daniel Humphreys

About the Author

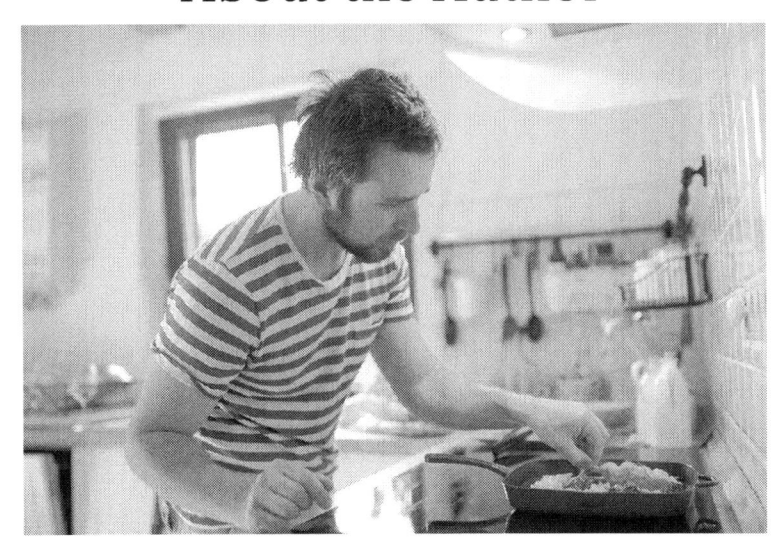

Daniel Humphreys

Many people will ask me if I am German or Norman, and my answer is that I am 100% unique! Joking aside, I owe my cooking influence mainly to my mother who was British! I can certainly make a mean Sheppard's pie, but when it comes to preparing Bratwurst sausages and drinking beer with friends, I am also all in!

I am taking you on this culinary journey with me and hope you can appreciate my diversified background. In my 15 years career as a chef, I never had a dish returned to me by one of clients, so that should say something about me! Actually, I will take that back. My worst critic is my four years old son, who refuses to taste anything that is green color. That shall pass, I am sure.

My hope is to help my children discover the joy of cooking and sharing their creations with their loved ones, like I did all my life. When you develop a passion for cooking and my suspicious is that you have one as well, it usually sticks for life. The best advice I can give anyone as a professional chef is invest. Invest your time, your heart in each meal you are creating. Invest also a little money in good cooking hardware and quality ingredients. But most of all enjoy every meal you prepare with YOUR friends and family!

Printed in Great Britain
by Amazon

78936803R00073